Ryan;
Know you are still a
little young for this book
but think you will love all
the info.
Have a happy and
healthy 2018
Denise

Additional Praise for
Younger Next Year

"With optimism, insight, and humor, Crowley and Lodge provide sound information and practical suggestions for living a healthy and active later third of life."

—ALLAN ROSENFIELD, M.D., dean,
School of Public Health, Columbia University

"Men apparently are reluctant to ask for directions, but can they resist advice regarding their well-being? I think not. Here is a book full of sound information, thoughtfully provocative, fresh and witty. And better yet, you don't have to be a man to find this book useful."

—JAMAICA KINCAID, author of *Annie John*
and *The Autobiography of My Mother*

"A powerful message . . . for all concerned with living long and well, a book in plain English that weaves the knowledge of medicine and evolving science together with concrete advice and a thoughtful perspective."

—HERBERT PARDES, M.D., president and CEO,
New York–Presbyterian Hospital

"We owe it to ourselves to know that we have the choice to age in good health. This book tells you about it. Read it."

—JOHN S. REED, interim chairman,
New York Stock Exchange;
former chairman and CEO, Citicorp

"*Younger Next Year* delivers the goods. Confronting the myths and realities of aging, it is a treasure trove of life-enhancing recommendations that prove the so-called inevitabilities of middle age are not inevitable at all."

—DAVID J. DEMKO, M.D.,
editor in chief, *AgeVenture News*

Younger Next Year™

A Guide to Living Like 50 Until You're 80 and Beyond

by Chris Crowley &
Henry S. Lodge, M.D.

WORKMAN PUBLISHING • NEW YORK

Chapter photos by Janette Beckman.

Portions of Chapter Ten first appeared in *Aspen Magazine*.

Library of Congress Cataloging-in-Publication Data

Crowley, Chris.
    Younger next year: a guide to living like 50 until you're 80 and beyond /
  by Chris Crowley and Henry S. Lodge.
      p. cm.
    ISBN-13: 978-0-7611-3423-7
    ISBN-10: 0-7611-3423-9
      1. Longevity. 2. Older men—Health and hygiene. I. Lodge, Henry S.
    II. Title.

  RA776.75.C768 2004
  613'.04234—dc22

                                                    2004055353

Workman books are available at special discounts when purchased in
bulk for premiums and sales promotions as well as for fund-raising or
educational use. Special editions or book excerpts can also be created
to specification. For details, contact the Special Sales Director at the
address below.

Workman Publishing Company, Inc.
225 Varick Street
New York, NY 10014-4381
www.workman.com
www.youngernextyear.com

Printed in the United States of America

First printing: October 2004

10

To Hilary Cooper, and to Chris, Tim and Ranie.
—C.C.

To my patients: for entrusting me with their care,
for being my most important teachers, and for the
warmth and fulfillment they have brought to my life.
—H.S.L.

Contents

Acknowledgments

First, special thanks to Harry. Everyone warned that collaboration is a horror and a collaboration with me would be much, much worse. Harry prevented all that . . . just would not have it. Our collaboration, and now our friendship, has been among the great pleasures of my life.

We have had a world of wonderful help on this book, but a handful of people deserve special mention. My list starts with Alexandra Penney, who "got it" the minute she heard the idea and helped me from there on out. Laura Yorke of the Carol Mann Agency went way beyond the normal agent's role to get the book launched. She is a great editor, a terrific friend and a super agent. Our editor, Susan Bolotin, also "got it" from the outset and was a genius at dealing with two slightly strong personalities and imposing order on a complicated book. Special thanks, too, to Lynn Strong, our copy editor. She has been at this for a while, she's awfully good at it and she has a major sense of humor, which helps plenty.

Finally, thanks to Megan Nicolay, person-of-all-work at Workman, who, among other things, drew the indispensable "Healthy . . . Dead!" charts.

A number of friends and loved ones read the manuscript, but the following were especially helpful: Jimmy Benkard, Terry Considine, Joan Crowley, Frankie FitzGerald, Hazard Gillespie, Emmett Holden, Fritz Link, Tony Robinson, Lorenzo Semple, Jim Sterba and Jack Tigue. My beloved sisters, Ranie, Kitty and Petie, all commented usefully. Eric Von Frolich, my cruel trainer, was a great help on my strength-training and aerobics chapters. Audrey at Sports Club L.A. in New York has struggled to keep me fit, at least until the book tour is over.

My children, Chris, Tim and Ranie, were endlessly interested, endlessly supportive, endlessly kind. They are old people themselves now—Chris will be fifty this fall—and they just keep getting better.

The book is dedicated to Hilary Cooper and with good reason. She got me started in the first place. She was unflagging in her support, intense in her interest and sound in her judgment. As with my life, she made all the difference.—C.C.

owe a very special debt to Chris for his unstinting generosity, for the sheer fun of our partnership, and for the deep affection and friendship that have grown between us, and to his wife, Hilary, for all her support. Thanks also to my colleagues at Columbia University and New York Physicians, my professional family for more than twenty years. I could not think of a better group of people to spend a career with. To John Postley, M.D., and Seth Lederman, M.D., who have been mentors and friends for a long, long time and who gave invaluable comments on the manuscript. To my brothers and sister, and especially to my parents, who were always there, providing editorial advice and unfailing support in every way, as they always do and always have. To Laura Yorke and Carol Mann, superb agents who understood this book from the start and who wisely sold it to Workman Publishing, where everyone we have met and worked with has been outstanding. To Susan Bolotin, an extraordinary editor, who was not only a true partner in this, but played the role of Solomon to perfection when Chris and I disagreed. Finally, to my wife, Teri, for all of her love and partnership over the last twenty years, and to our children, Madeleine and Samantha, two fountains of joy in my life.

Thank you all for everything.—H.S.L.

PART ONE

Take Charge
of Your Body

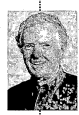

CHAPTER ONE

The End
of the World

So look, you're fifty-three, fifty-eight, somewhere in there. Great guy, pretty successful. Good energy. You're a serious man in a serious life. And besides that, you're in decent shape, thank God. A solid, weekend athlete. Well, fairly solid. Maybe a little overweight and the bike's been in the garage awhile, but you could get back there in a heartbeat. You're Type A at work sometimes, but hey, you get stuff done. You are one of those people who not only had the gifts to do all right, you had the temperament to use them. Good for you.

And a couple of months ago, you open your eyes in the dark and say to yourself, "I am going to be sixty years old! I am almost sixty!" You're awake the rest of the night.

Or you're sitting in the office and some twerp is looking at you strangely. Looking through you, sort of. As if you weren't there. When he leaves, it hits you, "That guy thinks

I'm a short-termer. He thinks this is the Departure Lounge, the little punk." You go around your desk and sit in the chair where the kid just was. An involuntary sigh. "Retire! What the hell will become of me?"

Last one: You're at a party. A pretty woman goes by. Not that young . . . maybe thirty-eight. And she looks through you, too. Just does not see you. As if you were dead. As if you were sixty. Same thing. That night, in the dark again. "Sixty! I am going to be sixty years old!"

In the morning, you suck it up, go to work. Do your job. Just like the last thirty years. But it's there, man. It's there all the time: "I am going to turn sixty. What is to become of me? As if I didn't know."

But guess what? You *don't* know. The point of this book is that *you do not know*. And you have the wrong picture in your head. You know what it meant for your old man and his father . . . for your mentor and a few billion other guys. But the rules are changing. Right now. And your prospects are different. *Quite* different.

Harry—that's Henry S. Lodge, M.D., my doctor, my co-author, my close friend—is going to give you enough of the new evolutionary biology in his chapters so that you can understand for the first time how your body actually works. It is going to be a revolutionary insight for virtually everybody, believe me. Once you understand it, and once you do some of the things that will seem obvious to you after that— why, you can choose to live like fifty until you're in your eighties. In your eighties, my man! We mean it. You may ski into a tree; that's a different story. Or you may grow a tangerine in your brainpan and be dead in the morning. Fine. But most of us really do not have to age significantly. For decades.

It is better than that. Most of us can be *functionally younger every year for the next five or even ten years*. That sounds like cruel nonsense or hype, but it's true. Limited aspects of biological aging are immutable. Like the fact that your maximum heart rate goes down a bit every year, and your skin and hair get weird. But 70 percent of what you *feel* as aging is optional. You do not have to go there. No joke. No exaggeration, even. There's a new, tough game out there. And, congratulations, you are eligible to play. You just have to learn how.

Here's what you think you know: You turn sixty and your feet are on the slippery slope—the long slide into old age and death. Every year a little fatter, slower, weaker, more pain-racked. You can't hear and you can't see. Your hips go. Your knees. And that great friend and amusing companion of your youth curls up and goes to sleep in your lap. Except when you have to take a leak, which is every half hour. You get petulant. Your conversation goes stupid. Your teeth are a bad yellow, and your breath isn't so great, either. You don't have any money. Or hair. And your muscles look like drapery. You give up. You sit there and wait. Go to the Nursing Home . . . get tied to a chair. Here's the graph:

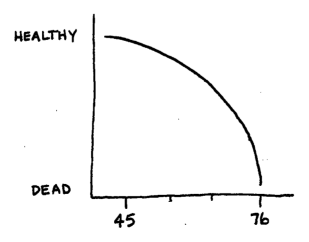

That can certainly happen. In this country, it often does. But it's a *choice,* not a sentence from on high. You can, just as easily, make up your mind—and tell your body—to live as if you were fifty, maybe even younger, for most of the rest of your life. If you're willing to send your body some different signals, you can get off the slippery slope. You can stay on a gently tipped plateau until you're eighty and beyond. There are guys out there skiing slalom races in their late eighties; I've seen it with my own eyes. And other guys that age who are biking in the steep hills outside Barcelona, where Lance Armstrong trains. Not just crawling along, either, like little old guys, but *doing it.* Going for it. Having a major good time.

And there are other old boys who are not interested in athletics but who are *still* in great shape and having a vigorous old age. So here's the lesson of the book: You do not have to get old the way you think. You can do all the same things, almost the same way. Bike, ski, make love. Make sense! Roughly the same energy, roughly the same pleasure. Roughly the same guy. In fact, if you're a bit of a mess right now, you can become a radically *better* guy over the next few years and *then* level off. No kidding.

At the worst, it can look something like this:

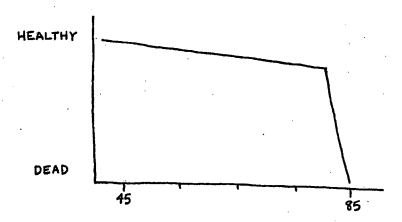

And for 95 percent of you it can look like this:

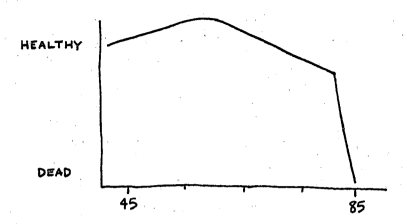

If you haven't been there, you cannot imagine how important the difference is between either of these last two curves and the one on page 5, because you probably can't imagine how bad "normal aging" is in this country. Take it on faith, it's bad, and the difference between the curves is profound. We are *begging* you, Harry and I, we are *begging* you to get off the slippery slope. It will make a fundamental change in the Next Third of your life.

Harry and I want this book to be fun for you. We want you to sail right through it before you realize just how serious we are. But let us have a candid moment. We are deadly serious. The stakes here—the potential changes in the rest of your life—are enormous. Think about the following numbers for a minute: Harry says that over 50 percent of all illness and injuries in the last third of your life can be eliminated by changing your lifestyle in the way we suggest. Not delayed until you're a little older. Eliminated! Along with all the misery, expense and lost joy that goes with being seriously sick or badly hurt. You may want to think about that for a minute. You may also want to think about the fact that 70 percent of premature death is lifestyle-related. "Premature" means before you're deep in your eighties.

Even more important, for me, is Harry's statement that some 70 percent of the "normal" decay associated with aging—the weakness, the sore joints, the lousy balance, the feeling crappy—70 percent of that horror can be forestalled almost until the end. *That is a huge difference.* I had some interludes of normal aging in my life, when my joints hurt so much that regular walking was painful and I looked for the cutout in the curb so I wouldn't have to step up three inches to get on the sidewalk. Think about that. Think about being so puny that you have to *rock* just a little to get out of a normal armchair. *That stuff happens. It will happen to you. It really, really will. And it doesn't have to.*

All this sounds extreme, but it is not. Harry will tell you about the emerging science to prove it. It is head-turning. I will tell you about the life . . . about me skiing like a maniac at seventy . . . long, scary bike trips . . . *windsurfing.* Caring about stuff. Doing stuff. About getting functionally younger than I was ten years ago. About feeling great, most of the time. This is not chest-thumping nonsense from some old buffoon; this is the demo tape. *Listen, you can turn sixty and get functionally younger every year for the next five or ten years.* So this is serious business.

What I Bring to the Party: A Report from the Front

My part here is simple: I have lived through my sixties, and I have been retired for a while. At seventy, I have absorbed and followed the message of this book for a number of years, and I am prepared to tell you the exact truth about the process. Mine is the report from the front. Optimistic, sure, but honest and unadorned.

And here's the good news. I have done pretty well. Not stunningly well: I am not forty. But I am, say, a reasonably healthy fifty. And this despite the following truths: I am an indifferent athlete at best. I am hugely self-indulgent (at one point I was forty pounds overweight). I drink almost every day and I am hardwired for pleasure. Absolutely hardwired. But once I got it into my head what the stakes were and how modest the commitment was—compared to the results—I was there. I did the "guy" thing that we all know about. I made a job of it. You know the mantra: "Suck it up, be a guy, do your job." Oh, and show up every day. That's the one thing we all learned how to do in thirty years on the job. Bring that edge to bear on these new commitments and you have it made.

Here's another nice thing: The *process* isn't bad. Some of it—the exercise part, maybe—sounds appalling and you'll think we're kidding. But it isn't and we're not. I wouldn't have done some of the stuff for a month, let alone years, if it wasn't fun, but mercifully it is. Slightly addictive, as a matter of fact. We'll explain. It's tough, but it's fun, and it works.

What Harry Brings to the Party: The Truth

Harry is the real McCoy. A board-certified internist (and a gerontologist), he is, at forty-six, consistently ranked as one of the best doctors in America in national surveys. He is the head of a cutting-edge, twenty-three-doctor practice in Manhattan and on the clinical faculty of Columbia

University's College of Physicians and Surgeons. He is also a serious student of recent developments in cellular and evolutionary biology. His is the report on that science—which has not yet made its way into the medical journals and won't for a while—and on what he has learned from his own experience treating patients in their fifties, sixties and beyond for the last fifteen years. The science is heavy, but Harry makes it accessible and persuasive. Okay, sort of accessible. But when you read his chapters, the logic—indeed, the near-necessity—of embracing his suggestions doesn't sound crazy at all.

By the way, the science is sufficiently new that Harry—a profoundly conservative man in this area—warns that some of what he says may turn out to be wrong as research goes forward. But not the basic themes. The revolution he talks about is here, and the science is real. He makes it clear that there are remarkable forces in your body—in your cells, all over the place—that are constantly at work, building you up or tearing you down. Darwinian forces—preservation-of-the-species stuff—that have everything to do with who you are and how you live. In his chapters (we more or less take turns), he tells you what they are and how they work. He also tells you how to manipulate and redirect them to your own ends. Like holding age at bay to a remarkable extent and for a very long time. Not completely and not forever, but a lot more than you can believe right now.

What you'll learn is partly what you have always known: There are tides in our lives that carry us forward or back. When you're a kid, the tide is behind you and you go forward, no matter what you do. Stronger, more coordinated, better focused . . . better able to understand and cope. But at some point the tide inside your body goes slack and the free ride is over. And then, in an instant, it turns against you. You get a little weaker, your balance is funny, your bones turn out to be frail . . . you can't remember things. And it begins to look as if before long the tide will be running pretty hard. And it's going to sweep you up on the rocks. Where the gulls are waiting. And the crabs. To eat your big fat gut. And your eyes. Take the guck out of your nose and your hair to make a nest. Go up there and eat you. Sorry.

But the interesting thing is that the tide is not that strong. It looks strong, because it's so steady, so remorseless. Yet it's manageable, in the sense that you can turn its relentless power to your own purposes. Like using the terrifying force of a wind that is rushing you toward the rocks to sail *into* the wind and safety. Harry is not a breezy guy, but he's awful smart and his stuff is worth a close study. All he wants you to do is change the way you live. Fundamentally and forever. Me, too.

Meeting Harry and Getting a New Start

I went to Harry because a pretty, redheaded skin surgeon named Desiree told me to. She had just taken off half my nose with a local anesthetic, and I was still crazy about her, which requires a certain charm. I had just moved back to New York from Colorado, where I'd gone to be a ski bum for a couple of years when I first retired. (I had missed that phase as a kid because I got married at nineteen and had three children before law school.) Anyway, I asked Desiree if she could be my doctor and she said no, but she had just the guy. Smart, decent . . . a terrific person. A WASP, she said, but not a dope, as if that had to be cleared up. He'd been her teacher of something in medical school and I'd like him.

So there I am in Harry's examining room, wary as a cat. Because (a confession) I don't like doctors. I don't like the haughty way they say, "Hi, Chris. I'm Dr. Smith." (I'm "Chris"? And he's "Dr. Smith"? What's that all about? And why do I always have to wait an hour to get this abuse? Lawyers don't do that. Doctors, man! And then the stuff they do to you!)

Harry has lovely manners and is a conspicuously decent guy. I am still wary. We've just been through all this terrible stuff. He's drawn gallons of blood, taken long, dubious looks in my ears and down my throat, asked lots of vaguely scary questions. And stuck his finger up my butt. Finally, it's the old "Why don't you put on your things and come into my office and we can talk a minute."

You just know he's going to say, "Uh, listen, I found a little lump up your butt . . . the size of a pomegranate, actually. Probably nothing, but there is some gangrene, so let's get you booked into the hospital and . . ." I go into his office, and no, he has not found the pomegranate yet. Actually, he says, I am in fairly good shape. Overweight but not bad. The fact that I get regular exercise helps a lot.

Harry is tall and oddly shy for a guy running this big practice. He looks at his computer a lot while he's talking to you. You wouldn't say nerdy, because he's actually kind of handsome, if you think about it . . . well, "nerdy" might cross your mind. He was an oarsman in college and looks it. But he dresses and carries himself so that I think "New England frump." Which, of course, is fine by me, because I look about the same. I once had a secretary who said, "Chris, you wear your clothes as if you hate them." Harry and I were cut from the same rumpled cloth in the same part of the world, the North Shore of Boston. We grew up five miles and twenty-five years apart. He drones on. Numbers, parameters. Blah, blah, blah.

Then, because I'm interviewing him for the important position of becoming my doctor, I say, "So, what is it about the practice of medicine that you like most?"

He stops, but only for a second, as if he'd been waiting to talk about it. "What I really like is the notion of long-term relationships with patients and keeping them in good health. Not just curing disease but promoting health, which is a different thing. I would like to help them have a better life, not just cure them of this and that."

Bingo! "What do you mean?" I ask innocently.

"Well, I've always been interested in aging as well as internal medicine. I actually got board-certified in both, although I'm not sure how separate gerontology is from internal medicine."

Then he turns and quietly drops the bomb.

"What I am sure of is that there is a fundamental revolution at hand in the way people age." He pauses and thinks how to get at it. "In the old days . . ." And he goes into the business about the slow, steady curve from fifty to death on the one hand and the new plateau on the other. Actually draws the lines in the air with his hand. "And you could be on the frontier of that change."

"Me?"

"Yeah. With your numbers . . ." He fools around with the computer. "Yup, this is pretty good. Uh, you don't smoke, and with these numbers and a more aggressive exercise habit, you could go on about the way you are today until you are, say, eighty. Maybe ninety. In fact, if you do a few things, you can actually be functionally younger. You're already in better shape than most of the men who come in here for the first time, but yes, you could be *younger next year* in all the ways that matter. Younger next year and for quite a few years to come."

I go over and sit in his lap. "True?"

"Yeah. You ski. Well, you can ski hard through your seventies. Slow down and eventually go to cross-country at some point in your eighties. Bike . . . you can do that forever. There will be a certain decline eventually, but basically you can be as athletic, vigorous and alert as you were at fifty until you're eighty or older. And for the first five or more years you can be functionally younger."

"What do I have to do?"

"It's hard to summarize, but there are three things." Did you ever notice how there are always three things? "Three things," he says. "Exercise. Nutrition. And commitment.

"The biggest one—and the biggest change for most people—is exercise. It is the secret to great health. You should exercise hard almost every day of your life—say, six days a week. And do strength training. Lift weights, two of those six days. Exercise is *the* great key to aging. This long slide . . ." again, the arching curve with his hand in the air, "can simply go away. Or go up for quite a while. And you can be yourself for the rest of your life."

I have about four hundred questions, but, uncharacteristically, I sit and wait.

Harry goes on. "Nutrition, too. You should eat the way you know you should eat but probably don't. If you possibly can, you should get down to your true weight. You're . . ." peek at the screen, "one ninety-four. You should be . . . what? What's your normal weight? One seventy-five?"

"One sixty-five, I guess. Maybe less. I rowed a little in college at one fifty-five and weighed about that until I was in my forties."

"Okay, if you could get back to one seventy someday, that would be great, but don't stew about it. It's much more important to exercise, regardless of what you weigh, and then learn to eat rationally from here on out. Quit eating the things that you know are rotten for you, like fast food and lots of fats and simple carbs. And eat less of everything." He says dieting is dumb and doesn't work, but that my weight would drift down, over time, if I exercised the way I should and quit eating junk.

"How about genes? I thought this was all decided at birth, and I could just sit back and take my beating."

"No," Harry says emphatically. "That is a profound mis-understanding and a lousy excuse. Genes are maybe twenty percent of it. The rest is up to you."

"Booze?"

He looks back at the screen again. "Social drinker," he quotes me from the questionnaire. "Two drinks a night." Then those lovely manners cut in, and he does not lean across the desk and shout "LIAR!" He just does the familiar thing about how a glass or two of wine is good but more than that is a negative. A lot more can be a real negative. Obviously.

"Commitment." He shrugs, as if to say this next part is harder to talk about. "What I mean is, you have to be involved with other people. And you have to care about something. Goals. Charities . . . people . . . family . . . job . . . hobbies. Especially after retirement, you have to dig in and take hold or things can take some bad turns." He stops, stuck for a minute, struggling a little. "It's specific to you. And it's awfully hard to generalize, but there have to be people and causes you care about. Doesn't seem to matter much what the causes are. They don't have to be important to society or make money, as long as they're important and interesting to you. There have to be people you care about and a reason to keep yourself alive. If not . . ." a little smile, "you'll die."

"That's it?" I ask.

"In a nutshell, yeah."

"Okay." I'm ready to go. "How much exercise? What do I eat?"

But that's the rest of the book. You're going to like it. It's going to save your life.

CHAPTER TWO

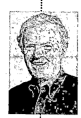

How's
Your Wife?

efore Harry gets his turn to talk, let me ask you a funny question: How's your wife? Or your lover or close pal? Whoever you got . . . whoever's got you?

How's she doing with the idea of your aging, of your retirement? Is she basically life-affirming or has she had about enough? Is she on your side? Or on your case? Does she like you? Do you like her? What do you think of each other, anyway, now that you're getting older? Okay, here's the real question: Is your union strong enough so it can be made into the foundation for the very different life that's coming at you both, at about a hundred miles an hour? Can you use the old stones, use the old beams, use the old love? Are you in this thing together?

Here's why I ask. It's too damn hard to do this thing alone, that's why. And it's a real help if you happen to have someone who loves you and whom you love. That may come as a little surprise to you. Some guys have a wistful way of thinking, boy, if I could get the hell out of here and get my mitts on young Suzie Q, *then,* by God, my life would begin. Or if I could just go out there and mess around for a while . . . just a few years.

Well, maybe. But I've got to tell you, I don't think so. I was single for a long, long time, and I actually loved it . . . had a fine, dangerous time. Excellent. Just like the movies. But that was then and this is now. I happen to know that this next phase—turning sixty or seventy and retiring—is a lot easier if you have a partner. And if your partner has you.

Look, if you don't have someone—or if your relationship is an absolute horror—fine. This book is certainly not intended just for married folk. There are other ways. Friends will do the job. Just one *close* friend does miracles. Networks of like-minded souls, too, especially if you're tied together by a passion for something. The great trick is to be connected so that you go into this next phase with some support. We were designed to function in packs. Strays get the sniffles. Especially with winter coming on.

Later, Harry is going to tell you some wild stuff about how mammals are actually hardwired to function in groups. How we have this separate brain for it. Weird but true. The disposition to work in pairs and groups runs deep in our bodies and our minds, and we cannot get away from it. So, let's go back to my question: How's your wife? Or your partner or your one close friend? And to our excellent advice: If you happen to have a decent relationship, don't piss it away in the vortex of change that's bearing down on you in retirement. You're going to need it.

It's worth mentioning this little point because a surprising number of men do exactly the wrong thing. A lot of relationships that have lasted thirty years or more suddenly implode when the players reach their fifties and sixties. People give up, just when those relationships could be turning into something pretty damn good. Perhaps because of the stress of retirement, or the pressure of suddenly spending so much time together. Who knows, but it happens. And it's not always a great idea, because this is a time when you need some serious company and some serious roots. A time when a lot of roots are being pulled out and things are getting a little scary.

I am an optimistic chap, and you should be, too. Much the best approach to life. But let us have another candid moment. Turning sixty can be awful damn bad if you don't watch out. And even if you do. Think about it. Some people actually *die* in their sixties. Not hit by cars or fallen off their bikes. Just die, of semi-natural causes. Like heart failure and cancer-of-the-this-and-that. It is highly unlikely that *you* will die, of course; I understand that. Especially if you do the stuff that Harry and I talk about. But death is out there somewhere, and it can make you moody. You keep hearing the waterfall in the distance, and you wonder all the time, What's that noise? As if you didn't know. Scary. Very, very scary. One of the basic rules of this book is this: "Be a guy; suck it up; do your job." Great advice, but it can be hard. And it's nice to have company. Preferably someone you know pretty well. You're going over the falls alone, babe, but it's nice to have company for as long as you can. Especially when you're lying there, listening to that cataract in the night. We are pack animals. Snuggle up.

Plan and Scheme and Get Ready

Harry and I talk a lot in this book about retirement, even though there's a good chance you haven't retired yet and won't for a while. We do so because it is such a huge deal and it makes plenty of sense to get ready for it as early as possible. To simplify our storytelling chores, we talk as if everybody's on the edge of retirement right now, or already retired. If you've got a lot of time to go, great. Our modest suggestion is to do something that no one does in this country: Think about it. Plan and scheme and get ready. Build new networks of friends and commitments that will be there when the job ends. Think just a teeny bit about building a new you—and a new relationship with your partner, if you happen to have one. If you're planning on working part-time or at something new—and a lot of you are going to be doing that—get your lines out, use your connections right now. Figure out what you're going to do and how to do it while you're still a player. Retirement can be a fascinating and life-enhancing experience . . . one of the most interesting and important things that will ever happen to you. But it ain't easy. And it's dumb to sail into it without giving it some serious thought. Okay, back to the story.

One of the basic reasons not to be alone as you head into your sixties is that retirement is so tricky in this nation. Science has given you another thirty years. Hell, forty for some. But not the dear old firm. They want you out tomorrow, and they're going to get what they want. With a terrible suddenness. From one day to the next, you'll go from being a critically important element in a complex social organism, a member of the pack, to being a guy on the street with a lot of shattered connections. Maybe you're a consultant or you go to the office a bit. But it doesn't matter, you're history. They'll mourn you like crazy for about thirty seconds, and then get on with their lives: "Jeez, I miss Old Billy. Can I have the rest of his lunch?"

"Of course you can, old boy. Here, I'll just take a little bite on the way."

As if you were dead.

That's hard. All that support, that whole network of colleagues and friends and enemies, the great flywheel of your life: things to do . . . things to be proud of or to fear . . . places you fit in . . . places you don't. All gone in an instant. And not much around in this society, with its nutty insistence on the nuclear family and faceless cities and no roots, to take up the slack. We should change the way we've organized society so that we make better use of the Next Third of our lives. We should foster commitments and communities that will last a lifetime, and I believe we will. Because it's so obvious. But not in time for you. American society has been rushing down this weird, atomizing, isolating track for a hundred years now—making us into rounder, smoother pieces for the global economy we're all so nuts about—and it's not going to stop on a dime, even though it should. So you're on your own.

Guys in this country *think* that's okay. We think we're cowboys and individualists who just happened to drop in to work for a while before we head on down the road. Dropped in for, you know, thirty years, but still the same independent guys we were, way back when. We think we have this inalienable core of individuality and solitary strength for the flinty-eyed ride into the sunset at the end of the movie. Like Alan Ladd riding off at the end of *Shane*. Guess what, partner. That was a movie. When the time comes for you to get on your horse and mosey off into retirement, you'll have a lump in your throat the size of Canton, Ohio. Where you probably should have stayed in the first place. And you'll be scared. The lucky ones will be saying, "What will *we* do now?"

I can answer that for you. For good or ill, you will invent a whole new life in a weird new world, *the two of you,* if there are two of you. You're going to build a new homestead. And it will have to last a lot longer than the rolling of the credits. In the old days, men could more or less count on dying a few years into retirement, but not you. You will probably last for twenty years, maybe thirty. *Almost a third of your life!* So the new spread better be pretty strong . . . pretty cozy. And homesteading is mostly couples' work.

If you happen to be blessed with a relationship that can bear some weight—or if you can retool and reinvent what you've got so that it can take the strain—then the great likelihood is that you two are going to be each other's primary resource for a long damn time . . . perhaps the rest of your lives. Primary company, primary joint-venturer, primary encourager or dissuader—the works. For an awful lot of us, it's going to be a huge part of the social structure for a while. The best relationship in the world cannot, and should not, be a substitute for everything you got out of your job. That's nuts. But it is going to be a primary resource, almost for sure. So start the emotional negotiations early. You are *real partners* now, whatever it's been like in the past. Talk as openly as you can and figure out who's interested in doing what, who can bear what loads.

And do new stuff together. Think, for example, about the heavy exercise program that Harry and I will be touting in the rest of the book. If there's a chance in the world of doing *that* together, or even some of it, it is way more fun and way easier. You may think, "Why, hell, she doesn't care about that kind of thing." Or, "She couldn't keep up." Maybe that's right. Or maybe not.

Give you an example, close to home. When my wife, Hilary, and I met, the gag was that she never went outdoors, except to go to clubs, and only wore black. We moved to Colorado, and she shrugged off that persona like Superman changing in a phone booth. In a heartbeat she was skiing, hiking, biking and Lord knows what. Not a real "athlete" by any means. Neither am I. But into it. And when we came back east and I got into what I call Harry's Rules, she was offish at first. But then she got into that, too, and we went at it neck and neck. All right, not quite neck and neck: I'm a touch crazier and still a little stronger than she is, despite her slight age advantage, but we do a lot of it together. A couple of days a week, say. And I cannot tell you how much better that is.

Think about it: six o'clock in the morning . . . dark out . . . time to struggle off to that wretched gym. It's *so* much easier if there are two of you. You go out together, you do it together, you come home together soaked in sweat in the freezing air. To the coffee and the paper. And you *both* feel great . . . pump each other up. Nice.

Or this summer at the lake in New Hampshire, where I've always done a bit of rowing. This summer, Hilary suddenly got into it. We're off, side by side, she in her Alden Ocean Scull and me in my Little River Whitehall. At dawn, usually, with the loons laughing at us, in still water before it gets hot. I often go farther, but not always. Mostly, we do it together, and I can't tell you how nice that is. Biking these days . . . same deal. No one would have predicted that ten years ago.

So don't be too sure that your partner won't get into the exercise stuff. She may fool you. Also, in the Next Third, there are important things that she'll be better at than you are. Making new pals, maybe. Keeping the children and grandchildren in your life, where you can do one another some good. Pursuing connections and commitments and networking for both of you. Those are critical areas where she may do the heavy lifting.

Hang On Tight

In a way, marriage in the Next Third is easier. It's like farm couples in olden times: less divorce and less angst because both players, husband and wife, had such important roles, keeping the farm going. Same here: you both have such important roles keeping your new lives going that, intuitively, you're going to show each other more respect, pay more attention . . . simply *care* more about each other than you have in the past. And by the way, that nutcase testosterone flood ebbs a bit. That helps.

Another candid moment. Some older men are suddenly tempted to take a sideways glance at their wives and think, Hey! There's been some mistake here. There is an *old person in my bed! I've got to get out of here!* As if you were so great-looking, you know, with your little belly there, and your stinky teeth. But never mind, it happens. There's a convention in our society that men age better than women. Not when they're dying, of course—*which happens five years earlier for men!* We don't look that much cuter when we're *dead.* But guys forget about that . . . think they're Paul Newman . . . gonna live forever. So, never mind that there's *an old man in her bed* . . . you've got to get out of here.

It is our presumptuous view that that is a rather cheesy sentiment. Probably a projection of your own fears about what's happening to *you* more than anything else, and not a good basis for action. We are not going to say anything in this book about divorce, young wives, and all that. Too idiosyncratic . . . too personal. But we do have an idea. Instead of sitting there, in silent, mounting gloom, thinking what's wrong with each other, how about embracing each other's vitality? How about a timely, resounding "Yes!" to each other at this critical moment, when you can both use it? How about taking stock of what's best and strongest about each other and *recommitting to each other's vitality*? Not a bad idea.

Having said that, there are limits to what your partner can do for you. You won't believe it, if you're in your forties and still full of yourself, but there is a real risk that you will try to put *too much* reliance on the relationship in the early stages of retirement. Men—even great guys like you and me—are a bit dumb about preparing for retirement, as I said. We go into denial and stay there. So, when the day does come, an embarrassing number of us turn, with something like tears in our eyes, and expect our partners to take up the whole burden of keeping us interested, loved, hated, amused. Sorry, gents, they can't. They cannot and should not bear that burden. Let's say they're nuts about you—which may or may not be true, after the rotten way *you've* behaved the last thirty years—but even if they are, they cannot shoulder that huge load and shouldn't have to.

You're going to have to work at connecting and committing to other people, other groups, to make your life work. You are going to have to exercise your charm, your persuasiveness, your ability to get excited about stuff and bring others along—attributes developed over a lifetime—just as you have to exercise your physical body. The more broadly and variously you can manage to connect and engage with others during or in anticipation of retirement, the better off you'll be.

But that's all subtext for now. The *black-letter rule* for this particular chapter is this: Get in touch with your wife or significant other or best pal, if you just happen to have one. Recalibrate, restructure and strengthen your deal, whatever it is. And head into the Next Third as full partners . . . homesteaders in tough, sometimes hostile new country. You'll have much better luck and more fun doing it together. Start with this book. Ask your partner to read it and talk it over. Use Harry's insights into evolutionary biology to trick your bodies and minds into staying strong for the next thirty years.

You're a couple of kids in an old Western, and you're going to knock over the Darwinian Casino together . . . live on the loot forever. She'll be waiting with the horses down by the river. Or you will be. And you're both going to ride for your lives. It's a romantic story . . . surprising after all these years . . . and you're in it together.

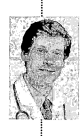

CHAPTER THREE

The New Science of Aging

W/hen I had been in practice as a general internist for ten years, I sat down and took stock. What I saw changed my life, the way I practice medicine, and ultimately led to writing this book with Chris. Things were going well. I loved my job, I loved my patients and I had wonderful colleagues. But the patients who had been with me from the beginning were coming into their late fifties, sixties and seventies, and things were happening. Some had become friends as well as patients, but most I saw only occasionally—once a year for their physicals and from time to time as problems came up. The annual checkups were like time-lapse photography, and in those jerky pictures I saw people I cared about getting old at an alarming clip. Many were sedentary, but even those who were moderately active were becoming increasingly overweight, out of shape and apathetic. And some were getting seriously sick. They were having strokes, heart attacks, liver problems, cancers and bad injuries. A number had died, and the timing did not seem to make sense.

One of the hardest things about medicine is delivering bad news: "We'll need to do some more tests" . . . "This looks suspicious" . . . "Why don't you sit down so we can talk?" All the euphemisms we use to say that life has suddenly—and irreversibly—taken a bad turn. I became increasingly aware that most of these conversations were happening long before they should have, and for reasons that were clear and avoidable.

It was not that I had missed a diagnosis or failed to spot something on an X-ray. I had done what doctors do well in this country, which is to treat people when they come in with a disease. My patients had had good medical care but not, I began to think, great *health* care. For most, their declines, their illnesses, were thirty-year problems of lifestyle, not disease. I, like most doctors in America, had been doing the wrong job well. Modern medicine does not concern itself with lifestyle problems. Doctors don't treat them, medical schools don't teach them and insurers don't pay to solve them. I began to think that this was indefensible. I had always spent time on these issues, but I had not made them a primary focus. And far too many of my patients—including some very smart and able people—were having lousy lives. Some were dying.

I had some further thoughts at that ten-year review. Most modern medicine is what lawyers and bankers call transactional: a one-shot deal. You blow out your knee, you have a heart attack, and you see a specialist. A short, intensive period of repair or cure follows, and the parties go their separate ways, probably forever. I realized that my practice was entirely different. I was likely to have long relationships with people . . . twenty, thirty years. That's one of the best things about being an internist. But that privileged, long-term look into patients' lives has put me on a different footing from that of the specialists. I am "on notice" of how my patients are living, and of how they are dying. I am "on notice" that the normal American way of life—and especially the American way of retirement—is dangerous and sometimes lethal. I am "on notice" that, no matter how great our medical care, we all need great health care, too—and very few of us get it.

It is inexplicable that our society, plagued by soaring medical costs and epidemics of obesity, heart disease and cancer, cares so little about these things. The simple fact is that we know perfectly well what to do. *Some 70 percent of premature death and aging is lifestyle-related.* Heart attacks, strokes, the common cancers, diabetes, most falls, fractures and serious injuries, and many more illnesses are primarily caused by the way we live. *If we had the will to do it, we could eliminate more than half of all disease in men and women over fifty. Not delay it, eliminate it.* That is a readily attainable goal, but we are not moving toward it. Instead, we have made these problems invisible by making them part of the "normal" landscape of aging. As in "Oh, that's a normal part of growing older."

"Normal Aging" Isn't Normal

The more I looked at the science, the more it became clear that such ailments and deterioration are *not* a normal part of growing old. They are an outrage. An outrage that we have simply gotten used to because we set the bar so shamefully low. A lot of people unconsciously assume that they will get-old-and-die: one phrase, almost one word, and certainly one seamless concept. That when they get old and infirm, they will die soon after, so a deteriorating quality of life does not matter. *That is a deeply mistaken idea and a dangerous premise for planning your life.* In fact, you will probably *get-old-and-live.* You can get decrepit, if you like, but you are not likely to die; you are likely to live like that for a long, long time. Most Americans today will live into their mid-eighties, whether they're in great shape or shuffling around on walkers. And that number is rising over time, too, so you may well live into your nineties, whether you like it or not. Which is good reason to make the Last Third of your life terrific—and not a dreary panoply of obesity, sore joints and apathy. "Normal aging" is intolerable and avoidable. You can skip most of it and grow old, not just gracefully but with real joy.

This was my epiphany. I thought, "I cannot, as a doctor, sit here and watch people I care for, and care about, go down a road that is leading them to an awful place without doing something. It is not enough to wait for the car to crash and then do a good job of treating the injured and dying." If 70 percent of the serious illness I see is preventable, then it's my job to prevent it. The good news on this front is that you do not need to wait for a presidential commission or a national health initiative to do something. This fight can be led, fought and won one person at a time. Starting with you.

As I have looked at the steady stream of people coming in for their first visit over the years since that epiphany, I have been struck by just how many of them suffer the downright *bad health* that seems to be the American lot these days. Not just older people, either; the horrendous effects of idleness and a rotten diet show younger and younger. With each new patient, I have the same talk I had with Chris, and if the patient is at all responsive, a new collaboration begins. The great news is that most people get it, and a lot of them have gone down the path toward getting younger.

Change on the Cellular Level

We are in the midst of a revolution in the science of aging. It is part of a larger revolution in our understanding of how our bodies work at the cellular level, and it has opened the door to healthy aging. The science behind this revolution is vast and extraordinary, covering fields as diverse as cell physiology, protein structure, biochemistry, evolutionary biology, exercise physiology, anthropology, experimental psychology, ecology and comparative neuroanatomy. Definitive conclusions from this research are still emerging, but the basic lines are clear enough that men and women from forty to ninety should act on them now. If they do, they can live radically better, happier, *healthier* lives than their parents, grandparents or anyone else in all of biological time.

Let's back up. Ten years ago, the basic science of health was unknown territory—the huge blank space on the map. But we have finally learned enough from studying disease to understand health. As it turns out, health is biologically more complicated than disease. In disease, the train has gone off the tracks and the laws of physics take over. The crash is terrifying and destructive, but the science is simple. Health is the reverse. It has carefully designed control mechanisms to keep the train *on the tracks*. The science of those mechanisms—the blueprint for our bodies—is phenomenally complex. Luckily for us, the controls are simple to operate. You need to understand only two basic, background points about the evolution of your biology to take charge of your health.

The first is that the human body is not a neatly integrated design package. The wonderful but wacky biological commune you call your body was cobbled together by nature from parts that evolved in different species millions, even billions, of years apart. Your opposable thumb, wiggling down there at the end of your arm, and a couple of extra pounds of brain are the only parts of you that are distinctly "human." Everything else is from another species. And don't think chimps here: We are talking bacteria, dinosaurs, birds, worms, gazelles, lions—the list goes on for pages. Your body, created with great optimism and fanfare by your parents in 1950, or 1930, or whenever, is mostly made up of cells whose basic structure and operation were developed by bacteria billions of years ago. The messages that run these cells are not the conscious thoughts that gave rise to the Renaissance or constitutional government. They are not thoughts at all. They are primitive electrical and chemical impulses that predate the dawn of consciousness by many aeons.

The second point is that you can control your deeply primitive cells with your miraculous, Renaissance-creating brain, but not in the way you would expect. You have to talk to your body in code and follow certain immutable rules. We're here to give you the code and explain the rules. Not our rules, by the way. Nature's rules, and you can't get around them.

Some Good News . . . With a Catch

You inherited a biological fortune. You have a stunningly good body, whether you think so or not, and a truly amazing brain. As a matter of fact, you actually have three *separate* truly amazing brains, from three very different stages of evolution, all working together. In simple terms, you have a *physical* brain, an *emotional* brain and a *thinking* brain. Although they are chemically and anatomically distinct (neurosurgeons can separate them like sections of an orange) and have different purposes, all three are densely wired together to get you through your day.

But here's the catch. Your body and brains are perfect for their natural purposes, but none of them was designed for modern life: fast food, TV or retirement. They were designed for life in nature, where only the fittest survived. Most of your body parts have as little business in a mall as a saber-tooth tiger. Left to their own devices, your body and brains will consistently and without fail misinterpret the signals of the twenty-first century.

Decay Is Optional

There's a critical distinction between aging and decay that you need to keep in mind from here on in. Aging is inevitable, but it's biologically programmed to be a slow process. Most of what we call aging, and most of what we dread about getting older, is actually decay. That's critically important because we are stuck with real aging, but *decay is optional*. Which means that most of *functional* aging is optional as well.

There is an immutable biology of aging, and you can't do anything about it: hair gets gray, gravity takes its toll and movies go to half price. Your maximum heart rate declines steadily over time, regardless of how active you are. That's big. Your skin degenerates, too, regardless of lifestyle. So you will *look* old, no matter what. But you do not have to *act* old or *feel* old. That's what counts. We haven't figured out a way to last forever, but aging can be a slow, minimal and surprisingly graceful process. And even on the appearances front, there is a huge difference between a great-looking, healthy older person and one who has let go.

Nature balances growth with decay by setting your body up with an innate tendency toward decay. The signals are not powerful, but they are continuous, they never stop and they get a little stronger each year. Chris refers to this as the relentless tide, which is a good metaphor. Whatever you call it, in our forties and fifties our bodies switch into a "default to decay" mode, and the free ride of youth is over. In the absence of signals to grow, your body and brain decay, and you "age." We may not like that arrangement today, but we are certainly not going to change it. What we can do, with surprising ease, is override those default signals, swim against the tide and change decay back into growth.

So how do we keep ourselves from decaying? By changing the signals we send to our bodies. The keys to overriding the decay code are daily exercise, emotional commitment, reasonable nutrition and a real engagement with living. But it starts with exercise.

You have to exercise all the time because it's who you are. More importantly, it's also who you *were*. What you came from, hundreds of millions of years ago. Your body is a gift from trillions of ancestors, and the fact that you're here means that every single one of them survived. Each one of them got it right; each one passed on a little more strength, speed and smarts to the next generation.

Our bodies and minds are precision instruments designed for succeeding in harmony with the natural environment. We are literally constructed to grow in good times—to be alert, to hunt, to explore, to work together, to build, to laugh, to play, to run, to heal, to love . . . and to survive. To do all this, we need our bodies and minds to be strong, active and completely in sync.

On the other side of the biological equation, however, we must allow decay to occur when necessary, because every ounce of body structure takes energy to maintain. Every muscle fiber, every scrap of bone and cartilage, every brain connection, every skin cell and even every thought consumes its share of fuel. Each has to contribute to survival and reproduction or it decreases the odds of genetic success. So in bad times, in stressful times, in drought, famine or winter, we are built to shut down, to hibernate, to retreat—to atrophy and decay as quickly as possible. From the point of view of the species, once the years of childbearing and rearing were done, this may have been a good way to age. In that mode, less food is used and, of course, death comes sooner to make room at the trough for the next generation. That's the Darwinian code for aging. That's how nature designed your body, and it's why decay becomes a little more insistent each year. It's circle-of-life stuff. Sound good to you as you head into those years?

Perhaps not. From an individual's point of view—from your point of view—there are problems. This is an appalling way to live, for one thing, and it does not make sense, for another. We live in temperature-controlled houses, not in an ice age, and most of us have far too much to eat, not too little. In the absence of paralyzing cold or famine, you might think our bodies would begin to adapt away from the semihibernation defense. But it was only a hundred years ago that we escaped those pressures—a staggering event in human development but a nonevent in evolutionary time. Our physical mechanisms have not adapted at all to the modern world of retirement, and they are not going to. Indeed, they have not changed one bit from the systems that were devised, over millions of years, to function in a knife-edge world where there was never enough to eat and always a surfeit of danger. Evolutionary change may happen, but not for many millions of years, so you may want to make other arrangements. You may want to come to grips with your old, Darwinian body right now . . . see what you can do to force some adaptation in your own lifetime. Remember, without your input, your body will constantly misinterpret the signals of today's world. It will trigger the "default to decay" setting. You'll start to deteriorate, to die. To understand why, we need to look at both the good times and bad times in nature, and how our ancestors adapted to them using the mechanisms and signals that are still part of us today.

Springtime on the Savannah

L et's start with the signals to grow, to get younger. It's springtime on the African savannah: a time of plenty in the place where we grew up. The rains have come, the grass is lush and the water holes are full. Predators are relatively few, and not a major threat. They demand alertness and respect, but not anxiety. Prey abounds, but the antelope, nuts and berries are scattered over a wide area, so hunting and gathering require hours of walking every day. Even today, Bushmen in the Kalahari walk eight to ten miles every day, foraging for food, with intervals of running and sprinting when they hunt. *That exercise—the physical work of hunting and foraging in the spring—has always been the single most powerful signal we can send that life is good; that it's spring and time to live and grow.*

In response to the chemical signals sent by that exercise, your body becomes lean, powerful and efficient. Excess fat becomes superfluous because the energy supply is fairly constant. Your body keeps a modest fat reserve to guard against hard times, but more than this is just a liability because lugging it around takes energy and slows your reaction time. Bone strength and joint health increase to handle the repetitive shock loading of the travel. Your heart and circulatory functions increase to supply the blood and oxygen to your muscles. The muscles themselves become strong, supple and more coordinated. Immune function increases to repair the ongoing wear and tear—the sprains, cuts, bruises and minor infections that accompany active outdoor life.

Your brain changes, too. As it gets these consistent physical signals from your body, it develops a chemistry of optimism: the ideal mood for hunting. Lab animals in similar exercise environments show actual physical and chemical brain changes, leading to increased curiosity and energy, an increased willingness to explore, increased interactions with group members, increased alertness and what looks for all the world like increased optimism.

Lean, fit, happy, optimistic, energetic, brimming with vim and vigor: these were nature's design specifications for you in the ideal environment—what you were built to be in the spring. This is the good life, and it's out there waiting for you. A life characterized by strong, aerobically fit muscles, a healthy heart, lean body, good bones, good immune system, high sex drive and an alert, inquisitive, optimistic mind geared toward working well in groups and building strong social networks.

We'll show you how to get there, but before we do, let's look at the dark side, at the way we live now. Let's look at our modern lifestyle, with junk food, too much TV, long commutes, job stress, marital stress, poor sleep, artificial light and noise, and perhaps worst of all, no exercise. Or retirement, which can just substitute boredom and loneliness for job stress and commuting. Springtime on the savannah? Not hardly. In nature, this lifestyle sends signals of deadly peril, and your body and brain make deadly changes in response.

In a paradox that you absolutely have to understand, endless calories and lack of exercise signal your body that you're heading into a famine that you may well not survive, and in response, your body and brain head into a low-grade form of depression. Ironically, in nature, depression is normal. It's a critical survival strategy. Let's look at real nature for a moment—not the beautiful sunsets, the songbirds trilling in the garden and Bambi and Thumper playing tag in the glade, but the killing fields. The nature where 50 percent of antelope foals are torn apart by coyotes in the first two weeks of life. Where kill or be killed is not a metaphor, but deadly real, every day. The nature where there is no margin for error. Not a small margin, but *none*. Adapting to good times is easy, adapting to bad times—to drought, winter or danger—is critical. Dead animals don't reproduce.

So, winter comes to the tundra. Darkness falls. Temperatures plummet to twenty below zero. Blizzards howling down from the north bring sleet, then snow—drifting to ten feet, burying food, driving prey into burrows, making it impossible to move. Most of what little food you get is burned up shivering just to stay alive. You start the long starvation of winter. As the months drag on, you wear down to skin and bone. The fat you built up over the fall steadily melts off as you battle cold and famine. You are locked in a slow race with death as you wait for spring.

What is hard for us to grasp today is that this was a regular, *normal* part of our human experience, and that depression-as-ultimate-defense lies deep within our bones. We used it every winter, and in every time of drought or famine. We survived by getting depressed. Not clinically depressed, or Prozac depressed, but survival depressed, as in let's slow down the metabolism, build up the fat stores, withdraw, turn inward, hibernate, cut everything back to bare minimum. Shut down and survive by letting all but the most critical systems atrophy and decay.

In fact, *all chronic stress works the same way.* Chronic stress, whether physical or mental, tells your body that the environment has changed for the worse and that you're in for a long-haul survival challenge. Low-grade depression combined with physical decay is your body's preferred state of health for this situation. The thing is, the signals for this particular state of health are pretty much the lifestyle of the standard American retirement: being sedentary, withdrawing from social contact and eating everything you can get your hands on. These are the primary signals of famine or winter, and your body will respond. With the unerring certainty born of billions of years of survival, it will respond to your behavior.

Being sedentary is the most important signal for decay. Your body watches what you do, your physical behavior, every day, like a hawk. In nature, there is no reason to be sedentary except lack of food. Remember that we grew up in Africa. No matter how plentiful the game, it rotted in hours. No refrigerators, no convenience stores, no microwave popcorn. You had to get up and hunt for hours every single day. The *only* reason not to go out and hunt was famine. Regardless of how much food you eat, that's what you tell your body every day you don't exercise. And on those days you're telling your body that it's time to get old. To rot. To get survival depressed—low energy, apathy. To store every scrap of excess food as fat, dump the immune system, melt off the muscle and let the joints decay. Time to find a cave, huddle in the corner and start shivering.

And this all starts in a heartbeat, because the decay signals get sent continuously, no matter what you do. That's the tide Chris talks about. Your body tissues and neural circuits are *always* trying to decay. Muscle, bone, brain: always trying to melt, like ice-cream cones in the sun. The good news is that the decay signals, though constant, are weak. If you don't send any signals to grow, decay will win, but even a modest signal to grow—a decent workout, even a good, stiff walk—will drown out the noise. Thing is, you need to do something every day to tell your body it's springtime. That's the key to this book. It isn't complicated, but you have to work at it every day.

Keep in mind that decay is not biological aging. Decay is the dry rot caused by our modern, sedentary lifestyle. Decay comes from turning on the TV when the sun is out. From cracking that beer while you watch. From every drive to a fast-food place to get a supersize order of fries or a soft drink full of sugar and caffeine. From riding around the golf course in an electric cart. From sitting home alone.

Decay comes from giving up on life and failing to engage. But decay can be stopped—or radically slowed— by using the Darwinian mechanisms we've talked about. Aging is up to nature, but decay is up to you.

The Brain Chemistry of Growth

Let's say you've decided to choose a "springtime" state of health. How do you get your body to comprehend your choice? Some of it happens automatically in your muscles and other tissues as you exercise, but a critical component is controlled by your brain. Not your thinking brain, but your physical brain—the one that came to you from millions of years back.

This brain is deaf, dumb and blind. Literally. Apart from smell, it has no direct connection to the world. Inside your skull, it is always dark, wet, a little salty and 98.6 degrees.

Your physical brain knows only what you tell it by the way you live your life. Your physical brain and body evolved in a harsh world, with no second chances, and their mechanisms are as fundamental as the orbit of the earth around the sun. Until the day you die, they will believe, with relentless certainty, that you still live in nature. That's why the way you choose to live your daily life determines your state of health—good or bad, whether you like it or not. Health is your physical brain's *perfect* adaptation of your body to the world it *thinks* you live in. This is not about disease, that's different. No one chooses disease. It's just plain bad luck, though often piled on top of bad health. But *you* choose your state of health. You can see this as a burden or a privilege, a gift or a curse, but you can't put it down and you can't get away from it. That's great news, if you understand the rules, because it's not that hard to take over the controls.

Taking charge starts with a look at how the whole system was designed, and that takes us back to the beginning. The first stirrings of life began 3.5 *billion* years ago, with our direct ancestors—algae, yeast and then bacteria. That pedigree is not humiliating, it's awe-inspiring, and we should be grateful for it. We do ourselves a great disservice by thinking we can divorce ourselves from evolution. Your family tree goes back 3,500 million years, and every second of it was spent perfecting the body and brains you inherited. Not one second of wasted time, mind you, but 3.5 billion years of making you perfect.

The Information Age

About half of your basic metabolic machinery comes directly from bacteria, unchanged, ticking along perfectly for millennia. These single-cell ancestors, together with yeast and algae, lived in a constant street fight where every cell competed for itself alone. All advanced organisms, from worm to human, have organized multiple cells that work together. The whole *is* greater than the parts, for the same reason that organizations are often more successful than individuals: communication.

Simple organisms communicate by leaking chemicals directly between cells. It's the origin of your sense of smell, which is your most primitive sense: the way the smell of coffee and bacon in the morning wakes up your whole body is a good example of how well it works. In general, however, the more cells in a body, the more information needed to make it all work, and as we evolved larger bodies with more sophisticated tissues, we developed primitive nervous systems, along with the blood-borne chemical signals we call hormones. As we continued to evolve, the neural and hormonal systems became ever more complex and adaptable, and allowed us to explore an ever-expanding range of biological possibilities.

Today, you are awash in information. You have billions of cells, and each one is constantly signaling its neighbors with highly nuanced chemical messages. Every scrap of tissue has a rich network of nerve connections and hormonal receptors, and millions of their signals fly around your body all the time. All the traffic on the Internet and all the phone calls around the world are dwarfed by the information traffic in your body.

That's not a metaphor. You send *trillions* of internal signals all day, every day, from the moment of your conception until you die. You talk to your body all the time in a constant stream of chatter, day and night, year in and year out. You won't, and indeed you can't, shut up. And all your tissues, every single part of your body and your brain—they listen to you, all the time. They hang on your every word, obey your every command. But they don't speak English. They read the language of your body. And you will shudder when you learn what you've been telling them.

The Language of Nature

Five hundred million years ago, give or take, our early invertebrate ancestors (snails and jellyfish and such) developed most of the neural hormones and brain chemicals we use today—chemicals very similar to Valium, adrenaline, cocaine and morphine. We didn't invent any of this stuff when we came along; we just bought it off the rack as we moved up the evolutionary ladder. It's true. Worms and snails run their bodies and nervous systems with the same chemicals and hormones you're using right now as you read these words.

It took another couple of hundred million years to get from worms to the first brain, but finally the fish figured it out. Salmon have the same basic, physical brain you do, or, more accurately, you have theirs. The fish passed it on to the amphibians, who spun off dinosaurs, reptiles and birds (more ancestors: it's getting crowded on the family tree), and they all kept refining that physical brain. Structurally, it sits right at the top of the spinal cord, sorting millions of inputs every second and coordinating the output to match.

We split off from reptiles two hundred million years ago, but we carried their gift, the physical brain, with us, largely unchanged, and it runs our bodies today. It's your purely physical brain, but what a brain it is! No feelings, and no true thoughts, but phenomenally complex physical reactions. It's a work of art, a miracle in its own right, an absolute treasure. Think of a marlin leaping out of the water or a hawk swooping down on its prey. The sheer athletic poetry of motion is a function of this brain. So put aside all your conceptions of fish, reptiles and birds as lower life-forms. There is not a single bird alive that you can match for physical grace and coordination.

Neuroscientists label this brain the reptilian brain, the hindbrain or the primitive brain. Each label carries with it the dismissive suggestion that this is some crude piece of machinery along the road to the perfection of our human neo-cortex. The reverse is far more accurate. The physical brain runs our bodies, and it does so with near seamless perfection. Try to use your thinking brain to ride a bike and you'll end up surfing the pavement on your face. Then watch old footage of Greg Louganis, spinning and tumbling through space in a perfectly coordinated free fall and entering the water without a trace. That's all completely automatic, not a thought to be found. It's the physical brain, and yours is innately as powerful as his.

Your physical brain also runs your metabolism, cease-lessly gearing every organ, tissue and cell to the immediate energy demands of the moment. Automatically monitoring every conceivable aspect of your physical being and keeping your whole body in a supreme harmony. That's why exercise is the master signal for growth, because it's the language of your physical brain. Celebrate this brain, and understand that it operates on some miraculous autopilot level every moment of every day. This is the brain that does *exactly* what you tell it to every second. This is your body's master control center.

You need to reconnect directly to your physical brain. You've shut it in the closet long enough. After days at the office, nights in front of the TV, this miracle machine is wait-ing for you to take it out for a spin. To *not* do this is a dangerous waste. Because there is also a dark side; there is also decay.

Life is energy. That's all that matters to nature. For 3,500 million years, life has walked a razor-thin edge between energy and exertion. Biologically, there is no such thing as retirement, or even aging. There is only growth or decay. And your body looks to you to choose between them. Fast food, sedentary lifestyles, modern stress, loneliness, retirement and old age have no evolutionary basis. Your physical brain does, and it is ancient and primal beyond anything you can imagine. Billions of years of life, but especially of death, have honed it to shut down nonessential functions with the ruthless efficiency of the shark, from which it came. And like the cold, dead eyes of the shark, this brain has no care for your happiness, no thought about your retirement. It is a ceaseless machine, in relentless pursuit of the perfect match between input and output—between growth and decay. It does its job every second of every day, whether you like it or not, whether you know it or not, and whether you take charge of it or not. With that in mind, think about what your physical brain learned from the way you lived today, and think about whether it told your body to grow or decay.

Stepping Out of the Crucible

The game has changed for us because we have luxuries and choices in our modern lives that have no parallel in our biology. In a remarkable triumph of ego over intellect, we simply assume that we were "made" for this life; that we were purpose-built for life in the twenty-first century. That is a deeply mistaken view, and one we must get over.

Unique among all the generations of living creatures that have wandered this earth for more than three billion years, we have stepped out of the crucible of evolution. We simply stood up and walked out of nature. Most of us are not likely to face starvation. We are not hunting or hunted. Life for us is not the razor-thin line between famine and plenty. From the point of view of shaping our species, death by starvation or cold has gone away. For the first time ever, there is enough to eat and no one capable of eating us. It is impossible to overstate the importance of that development or the depth of the change. Almost incomprehensibly, the great problem of our time is surfeit. And idleness. Our ancestors ran for their lives for hundreds of millions of years, desperately searching for food, storing it up in their bodies against the certainty of drought, ice and starvation. And then, in a twinkling, all that was gone and a fundamental law of creation ceased to apply. This is arguably the most profound shift, ever, in the way the world works.

Understandably, our Darwinian bodies and primitive brains are not going to catch up with this astonishing state of affairs. We live, in this new safety, in this new time of plenty, like drunken sailors freshly delivered from terrible peril. And sure enough, we have become ill. We forget our roots, forget our past, forget how our bodies and our minds were made, and we contract terrible and weird new sicknesses. Our bodies do not know how to "read" this plenty, and we eat ourselves to death. Our minds do not know how to "read" the absence of danger, the absence of the need to hunt or gather—the idleness. And we soften to death. Our amazingly effective hearts start to fail us in epidemic numbers, and in ways that have no parallel in nature.

In short, we have adopted a lifestyle which—for people designed as we were designed—is nothing less than a disease. Think about that. Our lifestyle—especially in retirement, especially in this wonderful country—is a disease more deadly than cancer, war or plague. We live longer because of modern medicine, but many of us live wretchedly and many of us die much younger than we should. The point of this book is that we have to learn to cure ourselves, or, in the midst of all this plenty, we will live and prematurely die in unnecessary pain—in bodies that believe they are in the grip of famine.

So how do we choose between decay and growth, between older and younger? We are not going to become hunter/gatherers again. Or even farmers, as farmers lived a hundred years ago, by the sweat of their brows. So, instead, we have to simulate a little of life in the survivalist world. We have to play on the physical stage in order to take control of our Darwinian bodies, and our minds, too—since they are so intimately wired together that it is useless to think of the well-being of the one without the other.

The take-home message is simple. Everything you do physically, everything you eat, everything you think and feel, every emotion and experience changes your body and your brain in physical ways that were set in stone millions or billions of years ago. Physical exercise and involvement in life trigger great waves of "grow" messages throughout your body and mind. If you send the right messages, you have several billion years of evolution and trillions of ancestors on your side, sending out primitive messages by the billions, making you stronger, more agile, smarter . . . better able to take hard knocks. Exercise is the only way to engage your body and your physical brain, but if you do it, you will get "younger." Not completely, but to an astonishing degree.

The physical messages you send by being consciously and steadily active, and the emotional messages you send by being engaged in the great hunt of life, *can override the default message*. With relatively little effort, you can mimic a younger man in his prime—exercising, interacting, making love—and your body will go along. Remember, the tide is relentless, but it is not that strong. If we are relentless ourselves, if we are active and engaged *every day,* we can resist and even swim against the tide into very old age. It takes work and routine, but that's what most of us have had all our lives. Bring those gifts and that discipline to bear on this new set of problems, and you can set the *realistic* goal of living like fifty until you're eighty and beyond.

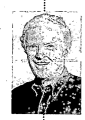

CHAPTER FOUR

Swimming Against the Tide

When Harry and I started, this was going to be a simple book. It still is, ultimately, but it gets a little complicated in places, which is why we thought it might be a good idea to have this one chapter up front to set out Harry's First Rule. One simple rule to learn (and follow when all else fails) before you get lost or bored or decide to go have a drink.

It goes like this: *Exercise six days a week for the rest of your life.* Sorry, but that's it. No negotiations. No give. No excuses. Six days, serious exercise, until you die. Well, if you're still in your forties and stretched to the breaking point with work, kids and travel, we can talk about four or five days, but six is much better even then. And after age fifty, six is mandatory. By then the tide is starting to pick up, and you need help staying off the rocks. In fact, my version of the rule would have been "Exercise *hard* six days a week," but Harry convinced me that that would scare the horses.

This is not an exercise book for geezers. It's not an exercise book at all. And it is at least possible that Harry's First Rule is not our most important piece of advice. But it is the *first* rule. Living up to it, and seeing the early results, spins your head around. It opens you up to seeing the Next Third of your life differently. It gives you the strength, the optimism, the flexibility to do the rest. It is the bit of magic that changes you from the tired old loser you might otherwise become into something quite different. Once you get this trick, you can do all the rest.

The notion of constant exercise seems crazy, but it's not. The *tide* is the crazy thing in your life. Think about it again. Here is this wack-a-doo tide, right inside your own precious body, that wants you to get old and fat and sick and stupid. Wants you to fall down, talk nonsense, get hurt . . . get the sniffles, get the blues. Wants to sweep you up on the beach, where the gulls and the crabs are waiting to eat your guts. *That's* what's crazy. Doing something about it is sane. Exercise is sane.

Don't think of it as exercise. Think of it as sending a constant "grow" message to override that crazy tide! Think of it as telling your body to get stronger, more limber, functionally younger, in the only language your body understands. Do it because it's the only thing that works.

Harry and I are not dopes. We do not think you're going to slap the book down at this point and run out the door to the gym. But we think eventually you'll do exactly that, which is why we are now going to tell you a couple of things that will help get you thinking the right way. In later chapters we're going to tell you exactly what kind of exercise to do, and how much, and how to use *your heart monitor,* for heaven's sake—more detail than you can bear. But forget that for now. For now we want to set you up so that you at least have a shot at starting what we recognize is a revolutionary regimen . . . a wild change in the way you live your life. Read this next bit on spec. Before long, you may want to take a serious stab at this life we're peddling, and this will be helpful.

Make It Your New Job

We urge you *not* to start gradually. It is far better to make a sharp break with the past and a serious commitment to the future. If you are at or near retirement, we urge you as strongly as we can to make this your new job. If retirement is a ways off, think of it as your first priority after work and do the best you can. But remember, as you get older, steady exercise rises on the priority list because the tide is rising. The tide has its priorities, and you must have yours. Or you'll be swept away.

There is one thing people learn in their careers, whether they're president of the company or mid-level what-do-you-call-its. They learn to go to work. Without thinking much about it, they learn a skill that children and heiresses do not have. They learn to go to work every day and do their job. That simple knack is one of the most powerful organizing forces in life, and you have it, etched deep in your conscious and unconscious mind. Nice going. Now use it in your new life.

One of the terrific things about the go-to-work habit is that it's a great prioritizer. Work trumps everything except serious illness or serious family problems. Daily exercise should be treated the same way. If you're going to have success with this excellent new life, you're going to have to give regular exercise that priority. Which may be hard. Some people have trouble thinking that exercise is "serious." They feel vaguely guilty about it, because it's too much like play. All we can say is, get over it, because that's nuts. Nothing you are doing in the Next Third is as important as daily exercise. If it feels like play, great; you're one of the lucky ones. But it is deadly serious, because it is keeping you from becoming a pathetic old fool. You think there's something more important than that? *Come on!*

Men are apt to be negotiators, and Harry and I are always asked, "Why six days? Why is that so important? What's wrong with three days? Or two? Or one? Isn't anything better than nothing?"

No, you silly son of a bitch! It's not better than nothing! Or, in any case, it's so much worse than six days for men over fifty that we don't even want you to think about it. It will sap your strength and drain your willpower. It will put you on the beach. It's six days because it *has* to be. Don't argue. Did it ever occur to you to tell your boss you'd prefer working two days a week? *Please!*

Actually, it should be seven. The tide is seven, and it's a boa constrictor. People think boa constrictors squeeze, but they don't. They just wrap around you and wait. You let out a breath . . . they take up the slack. Do it again . . . they take up the slack again. Until you're dead. The tide is like that. You relax . . . and it takes up the slack. So, no slacking. You're lucky that only an hour a day works so well.

May I say that I have not reached my seventies without learning a thing or two about human frailty and its corollary, the pathetic excuse. There will be days when, armed with a pathetic excuse, you will insist that you are unable to exercise. Fine. That will happen. But do not conclude

We're Moving the Middle of the Road

Here's another thing we hear all the time: "Yeah, but you guys are athletes. And this is nothing but another exercise craze. I'm no athlete. And I hate exercise. So this is not for me."

Oh, yes it is. Neither Harry nor I amounted to much as athletes when we were kids. We've gotten into it, thank God, so it's become fun, but that's not the point. The point is that steady exercise is *a coded message to your body*—and your mind—telling you not to turn into a dribbling old fool. Serious exercise, six days a week, is not extreme; it's the middle of the road. They just haven't moved the road yet. That's what we're doing, together. We're moving the road.

Early on, Harry said something that grabbed me: "In twenty years, failure to exercise six days a week will seem as self-destructive as smoking two packs of cigarettes a day." Two packs a day was normal when I was a kid. They finally moved that road, and we're going to move this one. You're going to lead the way.

that it's time to change Harry's First Rule. It's not. The rule stands. Try to get back in sync with it as soon as possible. Do not try to get the rule in sync with you. That would be dumb.

Jump-Start the Sucker

The best way to get into this new life is to take a deep breath, make a profound resolution and jump in, full tilt, for life. Do it as dramatically and with as much fanfare as you can muster. Tell everyone you know. Open a great bottle of wine. Whatever it takes. Because, let's face it, this is not easy. It's the most important thing you can do, but it's not easy. So improve your chances by making the beginning as big, as joyful, as solemn as you can. Don't decide to "try it for a few days." That won't work. Think about it hard for as long as you need and then jump in for the rest of your life. With ruffles and flourishes.

You might think about a "Jump-Start Vacation"—a trip where exercise is the central activity. For example, take a week off, you and your partner, and go on a bike tour in New England. Or Ohio. Or Europe, if you're rich. Doesn't matter. If you've really let yourself go in recent years, you'll have to work out some just to be able to take such a trip. But no matter where you are on the fitness scale, you can probably find a trip that will be right for you.

And don't think you have to spend a lot of money. You can bike somewhere near home. Or you can rent or borrow a cottage on a lake or the ocean and get a pair of sea kayaks . . . do that every day for four hours or so, and you'll really get a nice jump. Or hike in the Rockies or the Appalachians. Or go to one of the hundreds of cross-country ski houses in the east or out west; they're pretty reasonable and there is no better exercise or fun on earth. Or go to a spa . . . or a "boot camp." The magazines are full of them. But don't go to one where the emphasis is on herbal wraps and manicures; you want one with serious workouts and diets. Sniff around and find a good one.

A downhill skiing trip counts, too. Go out west or up to New England and ski for a week. Or two weeks, if you can. A month, if you can afford it. That's what I did when I turned forty. Took a whole month off from a frantic law practice and learned to ski, almost from scratch, at an age when most people are quitting. A little extreme, but it gave me one of my core pleasures, especially in retirement.

"Do not delay because you do not happen to have a bath . . ."

If it turns out you don't have the wherewithal to take a jump-start trip anytime soon, forget about it. Just begin. It's too important to let it slide, and it would be pathetic to use the jump-start thing as an excuse.

I came across a marvelous book in the funky 1890s camp where I wrote last summer, on a tiny island in Lake Winnipesaukee up in New Hampshire. Written in 1905, it's a Danish exercise book that was purchased by one of my grandfathers—an English professor by trade, but a bit of an exercise buff by incli-nation. It's terrific stuff, heavy on Indian clubs, photos of the mustachioed Dane in his undies, elaborate advice about the tremendous importance of baths. For some reason, the author was adamant about baths. Toward the end, he makes this excellent point: "Whether you are weak or strong, young or old, I advise you to begin with these exercises at once and rather today than tomorrow. . . . Do not delay because you do not happen to have a bath; you can buy one when convenient, and in the meantime be content to rub yourself all over with a wet towel."

So don't screw around just because you don't have the time or dough for a fancy bike trip. Just rub yourself all over with a wet towel and get going.

Incidentally, there's a lot of talk about skiing in this book, just because Harry and I both happen to do it. Don't be put off if you don't ski; most people don't. It's just a metaphor for vigorous sport. Anyhow, skiing counts, and you can learn it in a few weeks, whether you're forty or sixty. (You can learn cross-country in a day.) Try it. It'll be fun, and it will put your feet on a path you can travel with delight for the rest of your life.

One last thought about jump-start trips. These are the pre-lims, not the main event. The main event is the rest of your life. Take this book along. You and your partner can read to each other back in that cozy room at night. And swap ideas about what you're going to do when you get home. Plan. Scheme. Write stuff down. Start a notebook. Figure out which one of you is the planner and which the inspirer . . . divide up the tasks.

But get ready for what you're going to do when you get home. That's the point.

Join a Gym

A lot of you are going to fight me on this, but you have to join a gym. Doesn't have to be fancy—the Y is fine—but there's a structure to having a gym that nothing else provides. If you think outdoor exercise is ten times as pleasant and healthy as indoor exercise, fine. Join a gym anyway. You need it for rainy days. For winter. For the group classes and the weight machines. And to find the brute who's going to show you how to do weight training. You need a place to go, like your job. You may do non-gym things a lot of days . . . bike, run or ski. But there will be days when, no matter what, you will just have to drag your butt out of bed and go to the gym.

If you live in a small town with one gym, go there. But if you live in New York or Chicago or L.A., with a gym every few blocks, consider your choice carefully. First consideration? Probably money. Some of these places can cost an absolute fortune; if you don't have it, don't spend it. The simple places almost always have everything you need. Which is to say, a few aerobics machines and some weights, whether stationary or free, and an adequate, clean space in which to use them.

But remember, this is a priority in your life now. Bear that in mind when you decide what you can afford. Don't pick someplace nasty just because it's cheap, and then quit. That is false economy. Proximity counts for a lot, too. Getting there is more than half the battle. But it isn't the only thing. These places have their own peculiar ethos, their own atmosphere, just like companies or colleges, and it's important to find one that feels right. There's a beautiful gym almost on our block in New York, but for some reason it draws a petulant and depressed crowd. Better to walk a few blocks and go someplace fun. My general preference is for a place where there's a mix of ages and interests, with a slight emphasis on younger and cute. That's just me. You decide.

My wife, Hilary, and I just joined a place where everyone else is in his twenties or thirties. The facilities are remarkable, but let me tell you, even though I'm in decent shape these days, I still feel odd down in the locker room with all those young hard-bodies. There's an edginess among young male athletes that isn't relaxing if you're deep into your middle years. I've gotten over it, but I still think the ideal gym for men in their fifties and sixties is a place with a decent number of young people and some people one's own age. Not so easy for me because I'm so incredibly old. I hope this book will draw out gangs of people; I need the company.

But if you look so horrible that you can't bear to go to a place with lots of kids and gym rats . . . that's no excuse! There are plenty of places that cater to older people, and even more that do one on one, if you have that kind of dough. Me, I'd get over it and go to a regular gym, but tastes vary. The big thing is to *go*.

Even more important than the age mix at a gym is its spirit. Try to figure out if the trainers and staff are cordial to one another . . . say hello and stuff like that. The place should feel good. It's bad enough to have to go at all; it's impossible if the people aren't pleasant. Of course, you also want a place that has the right activities. Spinning, yoga, handball, squash, swimming, or whatever gets you going.

So shop carefully, if you have a choice. And remember, a lot of these places will insist on your signing up for a number of potentially expensive months, so read the fine print. Special point for retired folk: If you're going to be away for months at a time, be sure to check the gym's policies for suspending your membership. There are some rip-offs in this area. Last thing: Be sure the joint is clean, and the towels are decent. Gotta have good towels.

Excellent Tip: Try a Class

I find that classes or group activities are great motivators. My own favorite, which I don't recommend for everyone, is spinning class. This is a group of crazies on stationary bikes who race to loud music and manic exhortations from a class leader. Not for you? What about step class or aerobic dance? Take your pick, but try *some* kind of class or group activity. First, you're more likely to go, because there's a set time for class and that creates a certain discipline. Second, you're far less likely to dog it once you get there. (It's way too easy to dog it when you're alone.) So look around for an exercise class. One of them may appeal to you and it will be a blessing. What you want eventually, it seems to me, is a solid exercise *habit,* supported by a structured *class,* at a pleasant gym.

Hold the Presses for Fred Goldstone

Here's a nice gym story. On the very day we're to turn in the final draft of this book, I walk over to the gym at six-thirty in a heavy spring rain to go to spin class. I notice an old guy in class, pulling like a train. He's in great shape, energetic, nice-looking but old. Old like me. I speak to him on the way out. He is Fred Goldstone, seventy-four, a retired doctor. Turns out he's been spinning *five days a week, for seven years*. Does weights, too. I say he looks wonderful, and he says, all on his own, no prompting, "Well, it's interesting. I'm in better shape now than I was at fifty because of all this. Better than my sons, too. They're too busy. My wife's tied up this morning, but we usually do it together. We like it, but you have to have *discipline*." He nods his head and says it again: "You have to have *discipline*." So hold the presses for Fred Goldstone, a lovely, soft-spoken guy with discipline. Who is *younger this year than for the last twenty-five*.

Second Tip:
Pick a Time to Go to Work

One of the luxuries of retirement is that you can do this stuff whenever you like. But you know what? Whether you're working or not, it's a lot easier to exercise if you have a regular time. A time when you change your duds and head off to the gym. Or the track. Or the water. Same time every day, so there's not a new decision every time. For me, early in the morning is best. I can't sleep anyway, because I'm an old person. At six o'clock, I get out of bed and go straight off to class. Try it.

Here's some particularly boring advice. If you're still working and you're going to make exercise a priority, you might have to go to bed a little earlier. If you go to the gym at six, which is a great idea, you might not be able to watch late-night TV. Well, tough. Exercise is a priority. If you're going to live forever and be cute as a button, you have to make some sacrifices.

Harry can work out at the end of the day but not early in the morning. But give him credit—in a very busy life he is pretty regular. Noontime works for some. Instead of that big, fat lunch. But no matter what, pick a time. I still think early morning is best for old boys. The only real trick is to have a schedule and a habit. No one has the character to make the fresh decision every day to go to the gym. Go on "automatic" or you'll quit.

My Third Tip: Tap into a Passion

If you're lucky enough to have an athletic passion, by all means tap into it as a support for your exercise program. If it's an aerobic sport, you can make it your core activity. Running, cross-country, swimming . . . just do it. But even if it's not an aerobic sport, you can build your routine around it to give it focus and make it more fun. Don't miss a single chance to make this fun and close to what you enjoy.

Personally, I have the great good luck to enjoy a number of sports these days (ironic, when you think what a mess of an athlete I was as a kid). I love to ski, bike, sail, row, wind-surf and God knows what. When I sit on the hateful quadriceps machine, in pain, pushing that stack of weights up the ramp, I think of the bumps at Aspen or the steep pitches at Stowe. Sure, this is hell, but the payoff will be on those magic hills. And it will be worth anything. Pleasantly enough, a serious program of aerobics and weight training will absolutely revolutionize your ability to do other sports. The thought of that can keep some guys going.

Same with the biking. I sit in that darkened room full of spinning men and women, blazing with teenage music that makes my head hurt, pumping my heart out. And in my mind's eye I am biking along a pine-scented road, between stone walls up at the lake in northern New Hampshire, getting ready to climb a mighty hill. It doubles my pleasure. It keeps me going. Tap into your passion, if you have one. It helps.

So, you're asking, how serious is this serious exercise? Suffice it to say for now that you have to exercise hard enough, after the first days, to take up the slack. You will want to sweat. You will want to strain. You will want to feel your body getting traction. Not a walk . . . not a round of golf . . . not an hour in the garden. Don't worry about the details for now. Just know that you have to put a strain on the lines of your life so that your anchor will hold in that tide we talked about.

The Best People Hate Exercise

Some of the people Harry and I like best hate exercise and all its works. Men and women who live a life of the mind. Bookish folk . . . lunatic professionals . . . artists . . . gardeners. People who love to eat and drink and talk. And read in the privacy of their very own homes. They hate sports, hate exercise, hated school *because* of sports and exercise. And hate people like us who try to tell them how great it all is. They are never going to change.

Well, yes they are, if they will take their heads out of their butts long enough to hear a couple of things. Like: There is no "life of the mind." Mind and body really are one.

Besides which, from a Darwinian perspective, you most assuredly are an athlete. Never mind that you had skinny little arms in junior high school. Never mind that your hand-eye coordination was a painful joke and that you'd rather read than almost anything. You were still designed to hunt. In packs. You ignore that basic fact at your peril. You may not *like* exercise, but do it anyway. For your heart, for your mind, for your immortal soul. And for us. We want you around to talk to. Maybe we can go have a drink.

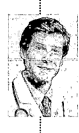

CHAPTER FIVE

The Biology of Growth and Decay: Things That Go Bump in the Night

iologically, there is no such thing as retirement, or even aging. There is only growth or decay, and your body looks to you to choose between them. So, this is the place where we take you backstage to look at that process—at the actual mechanisms of the new biology that has forever changed our thinking about aging. If things get mildly complicated, just remember that we are always talking about growth and decay. Come back to that simple point, and the details will fall into place.

First off, you may think your body is a "thing," like the Empire State Building or a car, but it's not. It's made of meat, sinew and fat and many other parts that break down over time and have to be constantly renewed. The muscle cells in your thigh are completely replaced, one at a time, day and night, about every four months. Brand-new muscles, three times a year. The solid leg you've stood on so securely since childhood is mostly new since last summer. Your blood cells are replaced every three months, your platelets every ten days, your bones every couple of years. Your taste buds are replaced every day.

This is not a passive process. You don't wait for a part to wear out or break. You destroy it at the end of its planned life span and replace it with a new one.

Stop for a moment, because that's a whole new concept. Biologists now believe that most cells in your body are designed to fall apart after relatively short life spans, partly to let you adapt to new circumstances and partly because older cells tend to get cancer, making immortal cells not such a great idea. The net result is that you are actively destroying large parts of your body all the time. On purpose! Throwing out truckloads of perfectly good body to make room for new growth. Your spleen's major job is to destroy your blood cells. You have armies of special cells whose only job is to dissolve your bones so other cells can build them up again, like pruning in autumn to make room for growth in the spring.

The trick, of course, is to grow more than you throw out, and this is where exercise comes in. It turns out that your muscles control the chemistry of growth throughout your whole body. The nerve impulse to contract a muscle also sends a tiny signal to build it up, creating a moment-to-moment chemical balance between growth and decay within the muscle. Those two same signals are then sent to the rest of your body. If enough of the growth signals are sent at once, they overwhelm the signals to atrophy, and your body turns on the machinery to build up the muscles, heart, capillaries, tendons, bones, joints, coordination, and so on.

So exercise is the master signaler, the agent that sets hundreds of chemical cascades in motion each time you get on that treadmill and start to sweat. It's what sets off the cycles of strengthening and repair within the muscles and joints. It's the foundation of positive brain chemistry. And it leads directly to the younger life we are promising, with its heightened immune system; its better sleep; its weight loss, insulin regulation and fat burning; its improved sexuality; its dramatic resistance to heart attack, stroke, hypertension, Alzheimer's disease, arthritis, diabetes, high cholesterol and depression. All that comes from exercise. But let your muscles sit idle and decay takes over again.

Exercise Is Healthy Stress

When you exercise fairly hard, you stress your muscles. You drain them of energy stores, and you actually injure them slightly. The stress of exercise is good, because it tears you down to build you back up a little stronger. You wear out little bits that need to be replaced after each use, requiring lots of fine tuning and minor repairs. This type of injury is called *adaptive micro-trauma,* and it's critical to your growth and health. It's the signal to your body that it needs to repair the damage—and then some. It needs to make the muscle just a little stronger. To store just a little more energy for tomorrow. To build a few more tiny blood vessels inside the muscle. To get a little younger.

The way it works is that enzymes and proteins from the exercised muscle leak into your bloodstream, where they start a powerful chain reaction of inflammation. White blood cells are drawn to the scene to begin the demolition process. These cells are the wrecking crew, the team brought in when you start renovating your house. The guys with sledgehammers, crowbars, wheelbarrows and dumpsters who tear down the old plaster and rip the walls apart to take your house back to its healthy foundation.

Since white blood cells are part of your immune system, you may think they exist primarily to protect you against infection. Well, that's part of the story, but your immune system's other job is to demolish big chunks of your body every day so you can grow. White cells are killer cells programmed to destroy bacteria, viruses and cancer cells by dissolving them in a toxic, caustic brew, like paint stripper. But they also use these same mechanisms to demolish the millions of cells that die their natural deaths every day.

With the short-term stress of exercise, this works well. Once the demolition is done, growth and repair take over. In a healthy body, the demolition actually triggers the repair process. That's a key point. The inflammation itself automatically triggers repair. Decay triggers growth. When the demolition is done, the plumber, electrician and master carpenter come in. New pipes, new wires and new walls go in where needed. The old stuff that's worth saving, the infrastructure and the detail work, is polished and sanded back to its original state.

Just remember two things. One: Decay triggers growth. And two: Exercise turns on inflammation, which automatically turns on repair. There's a carefully timed delay to give inflammation time to do its work, and that's when the demolition crews pick up the phone and call the carpenters directly: "We're all done, it's your turn now." Inflammation and repair, demolition and renovation, decay and growth—they're all ineluctably joined together in an automatic cycle.

The challenge for your body is to regulate inflammation in order to keep decay in a healthy balance with growth. If the stress is short-term, the decay triggers further growth. But if the stress is chronic, decay remains firmly in charge. Designed in our most primitive ancestors, way before brains were around to run the show, it's a simple arrangement that works beautifully out there in nature. The right amount of inflammation automatically produces growth. But too little—or too much—turns off growth, leaving only the background decay.

A Closer Look:
The Messengers of Change

You have two information superhighways in your body: your nervous system and your circulatory system. It may come as a surprise that your bloodstream carries information, but it does. Plasma, in particular, is a complex, living river of thousands of chemicals and proteins signaling and controlling virtually every aspect of your body: growth, decay, mood, immune function, cancer surveillance, fat metabolism, sexuality, joint health . . . and it all operates through inflammation and repair.

. Here's how it works: When your cells sense damage, say, from exercise, they automatically release chemicals to start the inflammation—to set the stage for repair. A few of those chemicals leak into the bloodstream, and those few molecules draw white blood cells to the injured area the way blood in the water draws sharks from miles around. After the inflammatory cycle has done its demolition work, the white blood cells go away, leaving behind a clean, fresh surface so the construction crews can get to work on the growth part of the cycle.

This chemistry is at the core of the new science we talk about in this book, so let's go into more detail here. The proteins that control inflammation are called cytokines, and they regulate every aspect of your biology. Cytokines are messenger molecules. They turn on or off virtually all the metabolic pathways in each tissue and cell in your body. Each tissue has its own specific cytokines, but they cross-react to coordinate growth or decay throughout your body.

Hundreds, perhaps even thousands, of cytokines are at work in your body, regulating growth and decay down to the most microscopic level. For the purposes of this book, however, imagine that there are only two cytokines in your whole body—two master chemicals that control growth or decay in every tissue and cell. It's a massive simplification, but surprisingly accurate. We'll call these chemicals cytokine-6 and cytokine-10, after the specific cytokines called inter-leukins 6 and 10 that control growth and decay in your muscles.

Cytokine-6, or C-6 for short, is the master chemical for inflammation (decay), and cytokine-10, or C-10, is the master chemical for repair and growth. C-6 is produced in both the muscle cells and the bloodstream in response to exercise, and C-10 is produced in response to C-6. This is your body's brilliant mechanism for coupling decay and growth. C-6 actually *triggers* the production of C-10. Decay triggers growth.

Now let's take a fresh look at the power of exercise to change your whole body in light of this new information. You have 660 muscles, which make up almost 50 percent of your lean body weight. Those 75 or 100 pounds of muscle are a massive reservoir of C-6 and C-10, a massive reservoir of potential youth if you do your part. Exercise triggers repair, renewal and growth by producing C-6. All forms of aerobic exercise produce C-6 in logarithmic proportion to both the duration and intensity of exercise. In marathon runners, the level of C-6 rises a hundredfold by the end of the race. It is an *automatic* measure of how much exercise you do, how much inflammation you cause and how much growth you will experience. In other words, how much C-10 will be released.

C-10 is key, because growth is the magic you are after. But growth is too complicated for neat description. Demolition is easy to describe, because, while it's important that you don't hit a gas main or anything, it's basically sledgehammers and dumpsters. But growth is blueprints, and master carpenters, and electricians, all controlled by C-10. We're not going to go into the fine details of how the cytokines actually do this because, frankly, it's too complex to fit in this book, but you will see C-10's effect as you build your stronger, healthier, younger body. The most important thing to understand about C-10 is that it is automatically turned on by C-6. Inflammation controls growth; that's the critical concept. C-6 peaks right after the marathon and turns on the cytokines that control repair, which peak an hour or so later and which stay at higher levels for hours after exercise, repairing your body.

At rest, only 20 percent of your blood flow moves through your muscles; in a trained athlete, that rises, with exercise, to 80 percent. Picture it: torrents, rivers of blood flooding through your muscles with exercise, picking up the cytokines, the messages of inflammation and repair, of growth and healing, and taking them to every corner of your body. From the top of your head to the tips of your toes. From your heart to your prostate, fingers to knees. Every joint, every bone, every organ, every tiny part of your magnificent brain gets its bath of C-6, and then the wonderful, rejuvenating C-10 each time you sweat. That's the right balance, good decay triggering growth.

Play the Music

This is important: Not all decay is good, and cytokine-6 does not always trigger the production of cytokine-10. When we are sedentary, the devil does indeed find work for idle muscles. There is a steady slow drip of inflammation, *but not enough to turn on C-10.* That explosion of growth comes only with the surge of C-6 you get with exercise.

Remember the old days, when you fell asleep with the stereo on and woke in the middle of the night to the needle going round and round at the end of the record? That faint *hiss-bump, hiss-bump,* filling the background silence? Almost but not quite inaudible? That's the C-6, playing in the background. The steady trickle of C-6 to every nook and cranny of your body all the time. No C-10, no repair, no growth, just decay. *Hiss-bump* in the middle of the night.

Another depressing point: You secrete more background C-6 as you age, no matter what you do. Dust in the grooves. Sad, but true. The tide sets against you. *Hiss-bump, hiss-bump* in the middle of the night.

Your brain is part of this, too. Chronic emotional stress also produces a trickle of background C-6. Loneliness, boredom, apathy, worry—*hiss-bump.* You can change this by being fit, or filling up your life, or both. Both is better by a lot, but let's stick with exercise for the moment. When you exercise, you get a high enough level of C-6 to trigger the C-10. You get to play the music of growth. It's not hard, you just need to become a daily C-10 guy. Exercise every day, at least enough to sweat, and you'll be fit, guaranteed. You'll be able to hike up a mountain at eighty, ski the black diamonds at seventy and outrun your kids at fifty, but more than that, you'll be healthy, more relaxed, more optimistic. Why? Because C-10 will automatically flood your body an hour after exercise like a sprinkler coming on at sundown.

C-6 and C-10 are just shorthand for chemical cascades involving hundreds of proteins in a dance of such complexity that we are just beginning to understand the details. Cell biologists will also tell you that inflammation is just cleaning up the debris caused by programmed erosion. Since the fine details of the mechanisms that regulate this will take fifty years to understand fully, we've used C-6 and C-10 as metaphors for the broader concept.

Researchers gave 10,000 men two stress tests, five years apart. At the end of the study, the fittest men had a third the mortality of the least fit. Think about that: one-third the mortality. And even more encouraging, those who had been sedentary at the first stress test but fit by the second—those who had turned their lives around in those five years—cut their mortality roughly in half. Cut your risk of dying by half . . . it's hard to argue with that. Even more encouraging, the benefit was on a continuum, so getting into better and better shape cut mortality more and more. For every additional minute the guys could go on the stress test, there was an 8 percent reduction in mortality. That's the good stress of exercise: inflammation leading inexorably to growth.

Stress on the Savannah

Stress, either physical or emotional, triggers a flood of fight-or-flight chemicals from your automatic, primal brain. When the lion jumps out from behind the bush, adrenaline floods your bloodstream and, through it, every corner of your body. The adrenaline triggers every member of the C-6 family and hundreds of other chemicals, too, in a surge that changes the activity and biology of virtually every organ and muscle in your body. Two things happen. Your emergency powers—physical strength, visual acuity, and mental focus—jump to their maximum intensity. The more interesting phenomenon is that all nonessential powers shut down to let your body focus on the danger. Your stomach, intestines and kidneys shut down. The liver stops cleaning your blood and dumps its sugar reserves straight into your bloodstream to give you that extra edge. Your immune system stops all background surveillance activity (say, for cancer cells) and gets ready to deal with the impending massive trauma. Your brain abandons long-term thinking and the development of long-term memory or higher cognitive function and focuses exclusively on the present. All muscle construction stops, bone construction stops, blood vessel construction stops, blood vessel repair stops. In short, in life-or-death situations, every scrap of energy and effort swings from long-term to immediate, from infrastructure to survival.

In nature, the bounce-back from this kind of stress is more vigorous than the decay was. (In other words, the surge of C-6 triggers a bigger surge of C-10.) So you grow a little stronger, a little faster, a little smarter, a little more alert.

In nature, life-or-death situations last only a few seconds. The lion either catches the antelope in a frenetic sprint or fails in the attempt. After thirty seconds of effort, the antelope is home-free or dead. It doesn't matter whether you're the lion or the antelope in that scenario—the chemistry is the same—but think of yourself as the antelope for a moment. As long as you got away, that was good stress. The shock told your body that there were predators, and that it was important to stay fast and strong, so when the adrenaline went away, and your body turned back to growth and repair, it did so with a renewed vigor and purpose. The same holds true for lions. They charge the antelope herd ten times a day, and they go hungry more days than not, but the adrenaline of a failed charge tells their bodies that they need to grow faster and stronger.

Our bodies *like* that. They crave the bursts of speed, the long trots to new grazing, the foraging, the roaming. Lots of alert but low-stress time, punctuated by bursts of excitement, and with a little danger thrown in. It's why we all crave a little bit of excitement. Daily variety. Adrenaline and C-10, perfect together.

But this positive message—grow a little better, a little stronger—depends on *daily* swings in chemistry. There is a chemistry of foraging and grazing, a chemistry of hunting, a chemistry of escape or capture. These are *daily* chemistries, the daily rhythms of life, and the messages are cumulative. Day in and day out, the messages accumulate, and every day that C-10 predominates, you grow.

Now we're ready to look at stress in our modern "advanced" lives. We have given up on swings in daily chemistry. No exercise, 70-degree climate control, too much to eat day in and day out, artificial light, but especially no exercise. So what are we left with? We commute in bumper-to-bumper traffic for hours at a time. We stress at work all day long. We go into deep slumps after retirement. We don't go back to foraging, we just run from the lion over and over again, and that creates a novel, modern chemistry of chronic stress.

Animals are rarely hunted into chronic stress. Changes in the environment do that . . . changes like drought, famine or winter with chronic C-6 and little C-10. And the stress of modern life sends those same steady signals for decay. Indeed, the levels of key chemicals found in our bodies today, such as cortisol, adrenaline and testosterone, are similar to those found in people who suffer starvation, depression, war, domestic abuse, post-traumatic stress disorder, chronic illness and other conditions where the *environment* is dangerous, or perceived to be dangerous, over long periods of time.

With the chronic stress of modern life, the chemistry of inflammation persists but the renovation never gets started. Decay becomes a career path for your body, and your blood itself becomes an inflammatory, caustic stew of C-6, carrying decay throughout. Not chronic stress as in two months of drought or four months of winter, but chronic stress as in decades of emotional strain, decades of being sedentary and overweight, decades of living in isolation. The tide is set against you. *Hiss-bump, hiss-bump* in the middle of the night, forever.

You can control the cycle. Commuting, loneliness, apathy, too much alcohol and TV all trigger the inflammatory part of the cycle. But daily exercise, joy, play, engagement, challenge and closeness all trigger the crucial repair.

That's why a man who's thirty pounds overweight, smoking a pack a day but exercising every day, has a lower statistical mortality than a thin, sedentary nonsmoker. Think about that image for a bit, because growth and decay also control the biology of heart attack and stroke.

It's All About Circulation

About sixty million Americans have some form of cardiovascular disease. Most of them don't know it, because it's preclinical, but it's there. That's the vast majority of Americans over fifty. It's been the leading cause of death every year since 1918, even during World War II. Being sedentary is formally classified as a major cardiovascular risk factor, increasing risk more than smoking or high cholesterol. Vigorous exercise, the real thing, cuts your risk of dying from heart attack by half.

Let's talk about the biology of heart attacks for a moment. It has almost nothing to do with our hearts, and everything to do with our circulation. Hearts don't fail; coronary arteries do. Arteries get blocked, they clot, and we die.

Our arteries are the one part of our body exposed to the cytokine-6 in our blood all the time. In nature, arteries never wear out; they never harden, they never clog and they never burst. In modern life, however, our arteries are exposed to the chemistry of inflammation, of decay, for decades on end— a steady bath of C-6 for fifty years. In response, they become weak and inflamed. White blood cells invade the walls of our blood vessels and sit inside, pulling down the walls, ripping out the old plumbing and, as an afterthought, absorbing cholesterol. That's what kills you, the afterthought. The absorbing cholesterol part.

Biologically, the cholesterol buildup is a mere footnote, a bizarre accident. Chronic stress alone won't kill you. It will melt big chunks of you, but it won't kill you. We, however, have taken it a step further, because we've coupled chronic stress with cheese and butter and red meat and chips and sugar and French fries. In nature, chronic stress is always coupled with starvation. The blood is caustic, but carries no fat. In the wild, there is no cholesterol to be absorbed. You are under chronic stress because you are starving to death.

C-6 draws white blood cells right into the walls of your arteries, and when you combine chronic stress with our rotten diet, the white cells turn into vacuum cleaners sucking fat out of your bloodstream. They grow to obscene proportions. They absorb so much fat that the actual cellular machinery of your arterial walls becomes invisible, buried under a mountain of goop. We don't even call them white blood cells anymore; we call them foam cells. In a renovation project run amok, the walls of your blood vessels fill up with all the junk of random demolition, held fast in a glue of fat and cholesterol. Over decades, this turns into the stuff called plaque, and plaque kills at least half of us.

Now let's talk about your heart. Your heart pumps blood out through a huge pipe, about an inch in diameter, called the aorta. The pumping has nothing to do with heart attacks. Your heart is also a muscle, which needs its own blood supply. That's where heart attacks happen: in the blood supply to your heart muscle, not in the rivers of blood it pumps out to your body. Blood comes into the heart muscle through two little arteries that come off the aorta. These arteries have even tinier branches, each about the size of a single strand of hollow spaghetti, that bring blood to your heart muscle. Shut off one of those spaghetti strands, and a piece of your heart muscle dies. You've had a heart attack. Shut it off high up, and it's a massive heart attack; you either die, or live as what we call a coronary cripple.

Biologically, your heart is a *simple* piece of machinery: four chambers, four valves and a little pacemaker. That's it, the whole thing. It's not the engine; it's just the fuel pump. $39.95 plus installation. It was perfected aeons ago, and it hasn't needed any refinement since. If your immune system didn't reject foreign tissue, we could replace yours with a dog, cow, deer or baboon heart tomorrow. For the average sedentary American, a cocker spaniel's heart would probably be big enough.

So what does exercise do for the heart? The answer is, not much. But it does wonders for your circulation. And it's your circulation that can kill you.

The Athletic Heart

Your heart will beat roughly four billion times over your life without a break. Not one minute of rest or recovery. You start out with your maximum cardiac capacity, and it's there waiting for you your whole life. It's your circulatory capacity—the ability to get blood and oxygen deep into your muscles—that changes dramatically. Your heart muscle is still virtually perfect today, a few billion beats down your life's road, despite your sins. But those small arteries are not. Even the arteries of "healthy" fifty-year-olds are coated with plaque that looks just like the topping on a cheese pizza. Medical students invariably swear off pizza after their first autopsy . . . for about a month.

Let's assume that you don't have anything about to pop right now, but let's also assume, without waiting for your autopsy, that your arteries have their share of pizza topping, a slight, subclinical blockage. Your stress test will be normal, but you won't be able to send quite enough blood to every part of the heart muscle that needs it. Nothing dramatic here, not true heart disease yet, just slightly less blood flow than the heart needs. Steady, low-grade secretion of C-6, but no C-10, and the plaque grows slowly larger. Pizza topping at autopsy, *hiss-bump* in the middle of the night.

If you ever have occasion to watch your own angiogram, you'll be astounded at how boundingly athletic your heart is. When it's full of blood, at the beginning of a beat, it's the size of a grapefruit. With each beat, it collapses violently down to the size of your fist. The coronary arteries, those little strands of spaghetti, are embedded on the outer surface of your heart, so they go along for the ride. They are coiled, twisted and kinked into half their original length, and then snapped back to full stretch about eighty times a minute. And this happens four billion times over your life.

The arteries are remarkably flexible and robust, but their walls become brittle as cholesterol plaque grows and stiffens over time. ("Hardening of the arteries" is a literal term.) At some point, as the blockages get larger and stiffer, one of the cholesterol plaques in the artery cracks. It's just a microscopic little nick on the inner wall of the artery, like the nick you get shaving with a blade that's a day past its prime. But it's still a nick, a tiny cut, and a little ooze of blood and rancid, inflammatory cholesterol leaks into your bloodstream from inside the plaque. The funny thing is that even though it's the inside wall of an *artery,* it's still a cut and your body thinks it has to stop the bleeding, so a clot forms right in the middle of your bloodstream. The clot grows to fill up the spaghetti strand, the blood flow to that part of your heart muscle stops and you have a heart attack. Decades of toxic lifestyle have caught up with you, literally in a heartbeat. That piece of your heart muscle dies over a few hours. The more inflamed your blood, the more the plaque is likely to crack, and the bigger the clot is likely to be. It's the biology behind the higher rate of heart attacks in sedentary people, in angry people and in people who have isolated themselves.

Strokes happen the same way, but since the clots form in the wall of the large carotid artery to your brain rather than the small arteries to your heart, they don't block it off at that point. Instead, a piece of the clot breaks off and floats up into your brain until it reaches an artery that is small enough to plug. That part of your brain dies, and that's a stroke.

There are two ways out of this deadly situation. The first is to starve the plaque of cholesterol with diet or medication. The inflammation remains, but it's much less deadly. You get old and weak, but you aren't nearly as likely to die.

The second escape route is to change the biology from inflammation to repair. Either exercise or joyful living will do it, but they work best together. This is the exercise chapter, but remember this biology when we start talking about how you live. Remember always that exercise and mood share the same chemistry. They work on each other and through each other. The "runner's high" is real, and it's both physical and mental. The chemicals of mood, arousal, excitement, fear, anxiety, optimism, lust and challenge are dumped into the bloodstream from the brain above, and the chemicals of local inflammation and repair are dumped into your bloodstream from the muscles below.

Calling Off the Double Whammy

Overall mortality falls with exercise. That is not a surprise when you consider that it's wounded blood vessels that kill you and that exercise heals wounded blood vessels. Blood vessels go to every corner of your body, and every one of them shares the chemical bath of inflammation or repair. Plaque in the arteries to your brain: stroke and dementia. Your kidneys: hypertension and, worst case, dialysis. Your penis: impotence. None of this is hyperbole; it's modern aging, and it's getting worse, not better. Of course, genetics and things like smoking and diabetes can accelerate the process, but underneath is the double whammy of sedentary, stressful lifestyle and dietary fat. They are the real killers.

The fact that exercise reduces death from vascular disease is not a surprise, but how about the fact that cancer mortality falls with exercise and lifestyle as well? It is now clear that cancer is an immune, inflammatory, lifestyle disease, just like heart attack and stroke. C-6 again. *Hiss-bump, hiss-bump* in the middle of the night.

Exercise changes all this because if, and only if, you exercise regularly, the chemistry of your blood changes. The chronic inflammatory signals of sedentary life get replaced by signals to grow, to heal, to recover. C-6 gives way to C-10. Remember, half your body is muscle, releasing floods of C-10 into your blood for hours after exercising, and your blood goes everywhere.

That's the biology of growth or decay. Heart attack gives way to health, death to life. And the bottom line? Exercise reverses the chemistry of decay. You swim against the tide.

CHAPTER SIX

Life Is an Endurance Event: Train for It

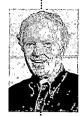

M an! C-6 and C-10, the Weird Sisters of growth and decay, coursing through your body, doing their mysterious work. Idleness as a powerful signal to decay . . . yikes! Exercise as the one great signal to grow . . . to live well. Wow.

All right, with this surprising knowledge in your brain-pan, you're ready to start thinking about Harry's Second Rule, which goes like this: *Do serious aerobic exercise four days a week for the rest of your life.* The first rule still applies, of course. You still have to exercise six days a week. It's just that four of the six have to be devoted to aerobic exercise, no matter what. (We'll talk later about strength training on the other days.) Aerobic exercise, as you doubt-less know, is the steady exercise that gets your heart rate up and keeps it up: biking, jogging, hitting the treadmill, speed walking and the like. It does not include doubles tennis and golf—wonderful sports and wonderful for you, but not aerobic. We're talking about steady, endurance activity that elevates your heart rate and keeps it elevated.

Eventually, most guys will be doing four days a week of aerobic training (at different levels) and two days of strength (or weight) training, but we're not there yet. For the first few weeks or months—and forever for some of us—it's going to be six days a week of aerobics. Most of that will be at fairly low levels, where you're sweating but can still talk with comparative ease. This is what we call "long and slow" aerobics, during which your heart will be beating at 60 to 65 percent of your maximum heart rate. (Don't worry about the details now . . . just take it easy.)

The reason for starting off with six days a week of long and slow aerobics is that most of us need, as a first step, to improve our ability to circulate blood around our bodies. More than any other single thing, circulation is the key to good health and to *doing* stuff. It controls our capacity to get fuel and oxygen to the muscles, where they are burned to create the power that keeps us moving. And—a matter of surprising urgency—it takes away the debris from the burning process. When you pant for air during exercise, this doesn't mean your body is desperate for more oxygen; it's desperate to get rid of the waste. Ditto the burning in your muscles: it's not from torn or stressed muscle fibers, but from the buildup of "ashes" in the form of lactic acid. Finally, circulation brings the blessed tides of C-6 and C-10 to prevent heart attacks and strokes, generate great mood and all the other wonders Harry talks about.

I don't know how you feel at this point, but I would guess you either want to close the book and watch TV or tear out the door and crank out a quick fifty miles on your bike. I wouldn't do either. The best move right now—and Harry agrees passionately with this—is to make a realistic assessment of the shape you're in today and then make a start that fits your condition. Start too easy and you'll get bored. Start too hard and you'll quit or hurt yourself. To help you position yourself, you might want to think about the early experiences of three very different men who started or continued exercise programs at Harry's suggestion.

The Man Who Couldn't
Walk to the Mailbox

Start with my favorite, John, a patient of Harry's who retired at sixty-five. At his checkup, just before he stopped working, John was a hundred pounds overweight. He had dangerously high cholesterol, high blood pressure, low energy, and he was eating mountains of garbage. He was under a lot of stress at work and at home, and he was sick with anxiety about retirement, even though he was not mad for his job. He was in dreadful shape and he was depressed. In other words, he was like a lot of American men of his age and station in life. Not typical, maybe, but damn close.

John and his wife were moving to Florida and got a place a block from the beach. Harry was worried about him and started talking about exercise. John wasn't having it. No, he said almost angrily, he was not an athlete, never had been one and had no plans to start now. Harry, in his understated way, said, "Fine, but there's a good chance you will die soon if you don't do something." John thought that one over and reluctantly agreed to walk on the beach once a day, six days a week, for a while. Give it a shot.

The first day, he walked about a half a mile and felt pretty good. The next morning, he felt as if he'd been hit by a truck. Everything ached, and he could barely get out of bed. But here's the thing. He showed up the next day. Tottered out of bed, God bless him, took a couple of Advil and went to the beach again. He walked about a hundred yards this time and went home exhausted. The next day, he did the same thing. And for several days thereafter. Soon he was walking a couple of hundred yards; then more. He felt like a dope, waddling along the beach out of breath, but every day he got up and did his job. In a few months, he was walking a mile in that soft sand, and he was feeling significantly better. He had better energy, took more interest in decent food and felt more enthusiastic and optimistic about starting life over down there in Florida. That daily bath of C-10 was working its magic.

A year later, John returned to New York to see Harry for his annual checkup. He reported that he was walking five miles a day on the beach, seven days a week. He had lost sixty pounds. His cholesterol and blood pressure were within normal ranges, and he looked ten years younger. He felt great. He feels great today.

Here's the obvious point: Don't feel like an idiot if you can barely stay on the treadmill for fifteen minutes at low speed the first day. That's serious for you, and your feet are already on a sacred path. It is not *struggling* on the first day or the thirtieth or sixtieth that's going to work. It's *showing up* every day and doing something. Do *something* every day for a week, and at week's end you'll be doing twenty minutes. Or thirty. Whatever. Push yourself a little, but don't push yourself over the edge. You get full credit if you change into your workout duds, go to the gym (or out on the road) and do some aerobic activity. The tide runs every day. So do you, if you want to stay young. Before too long, you should get up to doing forty-five minutes a day of aerobic exercise. Throughout the book, when we talk about doing a day of this or that, we mean at least forty-five minutes of actual exercise unless we say otherwise.

The Master Athlete

At the other end of the spectrum, consider Harry's patient Emmet, a serious endurance athlete who had done cross-country skiing and long-distance canoeing competitively. Emmet's wife was a serious athlete, too, and they had won a number of events together. Despite this history, their path had gotten bumpy by the time Emmet reached sixty, and he questioned whether he should continue his endurance training. Harry's answer was a resounding yes, and Emmet went for it with renewed vigor and determination.

For him, that meant a carefully structured exercise program, focused on a series of Masters cross-country ski races, which had him doing an average of two hours a day of heavy aerobics or strength training. And it worked fine. At sixty-one, Emmet came in fourth in his event, and he continues to train and race. He is one of the fittest men his age in the whole country. This book is not designed for guys like Emmet, but keep him in mind when you worry that maybe you're doing too much. You've probably got a little room yet, before you catch up with him.

Incidentally, it may be worth noting that Emmet had had some serious illnesses in his fifties, despite the fact that he'd been a big exercise guy all his life. You may ask, how come? How come a guy like that gets sick if exercise is such a cure-all? The answer is that there is a randomness to disease and death, just as there is a randomness to life. There's genetics, which matters much less than people think, but still matters some. And then there's rotten luck. But the point is, following the regimen that we're pushing enormously improves the chances of good health and a great life. I mean improves them by 70 percent. You don't get a guarantee—you still have a shot at picking up a fatal case of this or that—but 70 percent is not too shabby. There is not a pill or a course of treatment in all of medicine that comes anywhere near that.

The Man in the Middle

When I first talked to Harry, I was in much better shape than John, in better shape than most of Harry's patients, but not on the same planet with real athletes like Emmet. In response to Harry's urging, I took up spinning, which means joining a class of twenty to thirty people working out on stationary bikes to the accompaniment of music and the exhortations of a leader. I already liked to bike, and I had heard spinning was great exercise. Also, if I was going to follow Harry's Rules, I had to find something I could do every day in a manageable chunk of time. I thought spinning might be it.

So here I go. I am at the gym. I have signed up for a year at shocking cost, and I have gotten the spin class schedule. It's six-thirty in the morning, and I am feeling very, very shy. Because I am very old, I am forty pounds overweight and I do not look becoming in my biking costume. The instructor, an alarmingly pretty woman with a slight Euro accent, sees me looking helpless; she comes over to my bike and shows me what to do. The bike has a huge flywheel in front with a brake-like thing that can make it easier or harder to pedal. It's hard to get it started and really hard to slow it down. I feel as if I could wreck my ankle if I got off wrong. Maybe break a leg.

The room fills with beautiful creatures in their twenties and thirties. One or two old numeros, but no one as old as I am. The music starts . . . a din with a heavy, compulsive beat. The instructor has a mike, and she starts telling us how to pedal . . . how fast and with how much resistance. My hearing has gone to hell, but I follow as best I can. Speed up, slow down. Tighten or ease the resistance with a knob on the frame. I do not fall off, but I feel as if I could. And I do not break my leg trying to slow the damn flywheel, but I *know* I could do that.

"Out of the saddle!" the instructor shouts, and everyone stands up, pumping like crazy.

"Resistance!" she shouts, and everyone takes a turn to the right on the resistance knob. My quadriceps, which I thought were strong, start to scream. How many seconds can this go on? Actually, it goes on for about three minutes, but I don't. Did I mention that the walls are all mirrors? Well, they are, and I have just caught sight of my own face. I am so frightened that I sit down. (The instructors often urge novices not to stand for long.) My face is purple, a bad purple, and I am sweating in a way that suggests the onset of serious illness, not good health.

After that, I only do some of the things the instructor says to do. But I hang, man. I stay there until the end, all forty-five minutes of it. There are stretching exercises when it's finally over. My color is still peculiar. As I totter out of the room at the end, the instructor comes up and says, "Nice going. First time?"

"How could you tell?" I give her a wan smile.

She just nods and says again, "Nice going." I stumble home, bathe and go to bed. It is now 7:45 A.M., and my day is over. It is good that I'm retired; I could not go to work like this.

Okay, spinning was a bit intense, but the beauty of it—for a person of my ridiculous temperament—is that it caught my attention. It was *hard*. It was interesting. It was a challenge. And, with a touch of dread, I went back the next day. And every day for a long time after that. I've been doing it for years now, and I still get a kick out of it. And I'm in very, very good shape, at least for a guy who loves to eat and drink

Don't Skip This Box

You're going to get this twice, once from me and once from Harry. It is not pro forma advice, it is real. *See your doctor before you embark on any of this.* It is possible, at your age, that you have a condition you're totally unaware of that could make a sudden, new exercise program a grave threat. Don't take the chance. By now, you should be seeing your doctor once a year anyway. Do it before you start a serious exercise regimen.

In the same vein, let me join Harry in urging you not to overdo it on the first day. I did, but I am a bit of a wack-a-doo and have to take extreme measures not to be bored. Harry has a lot of war stories about people who went nuts on the first day and were knocked out for a week. Or never went back. Remember, the name of the book is *Younger Next Year,* not *Younger Tomorrow.* Feel your way. You are a slightly old boy now. You have Blacky Carbon and Gummy Sludge in your circulatory system. And your muscles and joints are not ready to go full bore. Take it easy. Sounds banal, but it's good advice.

and is congenitally unathletic. I sometimes feel guilty for not doing more, but from Harry's more rational perspective, I am one of the success stories. He says I've probably achieved about 70 percent of my potential fitness (as opposed to John, who is near 95 percent or Lance Armstrong, who is 100 percent), but that's fine. That's as far as I'm going. I can do everything I want to, and I feel great almost all the time. Gotta love that.

The point of all this is that there is a range of approaches to aerobics. I do not urge you to go out and push yourself to the point of purple on the first day, and Harry is appalled by the idea. But I do urge you to get into pretty heavy aerobics eventually. Remember, that walk in the sand in Florida was heavy for John. You have to do what's heavy *for you*. My early spin regimen would have been too easy for Emmet, too hard for most Americans in their sixties and near-fatal for John.

Harry and I are now of one mind on how to start. Start slow. Slower than feels good. But hold at that level only until you get your feet under you. Take it up as you get more comfortable. Feel your way, but eventually give yourself a little push. Don't go so slow that you get bored. Get heavy *for you,* but only after you've been at it for a few weeks and feel comfortable. You'll know.

So, What Kind of Aerobic Exercise?

The menu of aerobic activities is long and pleasant, and it doesn't make any difference which ones you choose, as long as you like them. Or can bear them. If you have some favorites, start with those. If not, here are some thoughts.

A surprising number of people like the endurance machines at the gym . . . the treadmills, elliptical machines, stair climbers, skiing machines and the like. This may make sense, especially in the early stages. They're easy to use, it's easy to regulate the "dosage" and the process is bearable for most. You can wear headphones and listen to music or watch TV, which helps a lot of people. The best one for me is the elliptical machine, with moving arms as well as feet, so I get both upper- and lower-body exercise.

The simple treadmill seems to be the most popular, which is fine. A hint: I think you do best to crank the *angle* of the treadmill way up and get your exercise by "walking up a steep hill," rather than trying to trot or run on the flat. Better workout for your leg muscles, less jarring on your joints, and you get a serious cardio workout much sooner.

Rowing machines are great, but only about seven people in the country have the sterling character necessary to keep them up long enough to do any good. If you're one of the magnificent seven, excellent. Same thing on cross-country ski machines: NordicTrak is a great workout for the people who can keep it up (including the endlessly virtuous Harry), but I cannot, even though I love cross-country.

Running is fine if you're up to it. Most men my age tell me their joints cannot take it, but there are plenty of lucky exceptions. If you try it after years away, go at it carefully to improve your chances. Do as little as fifteen minutes the first day. Hurting your knees or your shins or ankles at this stage is the work of minutes, but the consequences last for months or years. I hurt my Achilles tendon riding on a damaged bike in 1982 when I was forty-seven. It took me a year to get back into biking, and I couldn't run until 2004. Tendons are a slow heal. Being bored is much better than getting banged up and quitting. Run every other day. Or even every third day. Do something else in between. And continue to go slower than feels natural. This is not to say you should dog it forever. Eventually, you'll want to get a heart monitor and make sure that you're doing it hard enough. But not the first week or two.

Take Up One of the Healing Sports

Let me give a brief, heartfelt plug at this point to the blessed . . . the heavenly . . . the *healing* sports. Some sports, like tennis, pull you apart because they're centrifugal. Others, like running, beat on your joints remorselessly. But a few actually knit you together. Your muscles and especially your joints feel *better* when you're done than when you began. Biking is peculiarly like that. Swimming, cross-country skiing and rowing, too. They are the healing sports, and you ought to have at least one of them in your repertoire.

There is no machine more beautiful, more perfect in the form-follows-function line, more ideally suited to your purpose than the bicycle. In my thirties, after getting divorced, I kept my bike on the mantelpiece, the only piece of art in a dismal little apartment . . . a symbol of virtue and beauty in a chaotic life. New bikes—the composite/graphite beauties, the titanium jewels—are miraculously improved over the models of only fifteen or twenty years ago. If you're rich, run right out the door now and get one. But you don't have to. You can get a super road bike, with modern gearing and brakes, for a few hundred bucks. If you're more or less a beginner, you may want to get a "combination" bike; it's more comfortable and doesn't cost much, either.

Three other biking points. 1) You already know how to do it. 2) It's wildly good for you. 3) It's great for your legs. Later on, we make the point that building up your legs is particularly

A Word About Bikes and Safety

If you haven't biked for a while, you may want to remind yourself that you are fifty or sixty, not twenty, and that you have to be a hair more cautious. Wear a helmet all the time. I still bike in New York City traffic, but frankly, it's starting to scare me and I don't think it's a great idea. In fact, if you're just getting back into the sport, I'd start someplace pretty calm and bucolic. And, as with skiing or any "movement" sport, look around a lot more than you used to. Most important in biking and skiing: Be predictable. Go in predictable lines, and don't veer off without making damn sure there is no one behind you. You want to have fun, but you want to come home, too.

important in the Next Third. Failing legs are what can put you in the walker or in the chair. When in doubt, default to exercise that helps your legs. Like bicycling.

Or go swimming. It's cheap and easy to do. And if you go at it with some energy, it's great aerobic exercise. Swim fans often say it's the perfect exercise, and we can see why. You use almost every muscle in your body, it's aerobically demanding and it also stretches you out in a healthy way, like yoga. You see swimmers' bodies and think, hey, that's perfect . . . just what I want for the Next Third. My son Tim, who was once a bit of a triathlete, used to combine a weights workout with a half-hour swim. He says a half-hour swim is a *very* serious aerobic workout, all by itself, and the combination is ideal. If you really get into it, there are Masters race organizations all over the country. And the equipment consists of a Speedo and a pair of goggles. If you don't look so great in the Speedo, just keep your goggles on.

If you're anywhere near snow, do not miss cross-country skiing. Even if you've never done it before. For one thing, it's bone-easy. After exactly one day you'll be doing fine. It *is* a species of walking, after all. And once you get the hang of it, you can give yourself a massive dose of the very best aerobic exercise there is in some of the most beautiful places in the world. There is nothing better on earth than sliding gracefully along, under trees heavily laden with fresh snow, up a rise in the Rockies . . . down a country road in Vermont . . . over the golf course in your hometown. The only sound the hiss of your own sweet skis. Sneak off alone and try it. You will thank me for the rest of your days.

Of course, that first trip to the gym may not be a congenial one. After all, you're probably not in sensational shape. And it is at least possible that you are a big fat piggy. You may not look your best in gym clothes. (I weighed a slobbery 200

Start Out Long and Slow

In the next two chapters, we'll crank it up a bit, but for now just stick with "long and slow"—the pace at which you're breathing pretty heavily and sweating some but not killing yourself. You can talk while you're doing it, and you can keep it up almost indefinitely, once you're in decent shape. Pick your activity and go do it for twenty or thirty or forty-five minutes a day for a week or so. Or a month. However long it takes to feel okay.

when I really got into all this and looked nasty.) And, of course, you are slightly old. This may be your "new job," as Harry and I insist, but the gym sure doesn't look like the office. You don't know your way around, you don't know how to behave and you're probably a bit of a loser by local standards, whatever the hell they are. The people are intimidating. Almost all of them are much younger, for one thing. And some of them are absolute gym rats . . . in great shape and proud as peacocks. You have the strong feeling that they're looking at you funny. Or with contempt.

Well, the hell with 'em. You are not there to make friends or get laid. You are there to save your life. *So suck it up, be a guy . . . do your job.* Think about John on the beach the first day and where he is now. And if it really drives you nuts, let me tell you that it will go away soon. For one thing, in all the gyms I've gone to there is a genuine interest in and appreciation of men in their fifties and sixties and beyond who are Out There. The vainest and most self-centered gym rat in the world realizes, at some dim level, that there will come a time when he too is an old boy. And he only *prays* that he will be one of the lucky ones who are still working out.

A Dog Walking on His Hind Legs

I cannot tell you how many times in the last decade some nice kid has come up to me in the gym or biking or on the slopes and said, "Man, I hope I'm doing that when I'm your age. Nice going!" They're interested and want to know how you do it. Could they possibly get their old man to do it? And you do not have to be wonderful to pick up some admiration at our age. It's like a dog walking on his hind legs: the fact that he does it at all is terrific . . . never mind if he's graceful. So put on your skimpy, flesh-filled costume and go out the door. You are already a great guy.

Lying, Self-Abuse and Related Problems

One of the great barriers to success in this business is lying. People lie to themselves about what they're doing. They are absolutely delusional. They insist that their endless minutes walking to the john or whatever are all the workout anyone needs. Or the many, wonderful hours they spend with their dear friends on the golf course . . . sometimes even carrying their very own bags, God bless them. Well, that's nonsense. Golf is wonderful, but it's not aerobic. Quit lying to yourself and sweat. You've got to get out there and *do stuff*.

I talk to people about this book all the time, and the single constant in all those conversations—with men or women, young or old—is that almost at once the person I'm talking to starts to tell me about his or her own exercise regimen and how wonderful it and they are. It's ridiculous. These are big, fat people who have to take a deep breath in the middle of each sentence. Hopelessly face-puffed pudgies who obviously couldn't run a step and will be dying later in the day. People in such hideously bad shape, it's scary. They all tell me that they agree entirely about exercise and they are already hard at it. Well, that is nonsense! Outrageous nonsense! Please, please, please, whatever you tell me, whatever you tell your wife, whatever you tell your God . . . *quit lying to yourself!* You are not doing anywhere near enough if you're fat as butter. If you're short of breath. If you look like hell. Do not lie! You are getting in your own way.

Here's an interesting aside from Harry. For years, there was this neat little anomaly in how hard people said they worked out and their mortality. In surveys, there was a clear correlation between how much *men* said they worked out and how early they died. Agreeably enough, the results went: Work out more, die later. But for *women,* there was no correlation at all. Weird. So they did tests to correlate actual fitness, as measured by stress tests, and mortality. This time, there was a near perfect correlation for men and women. How come? Women lied more about how much they worked out.

Men lied some. Women lied a lot. Just tuck that away, boys and girls, and listen to me later when I tell you to go get a heart monitor. Both of you.

A Word to the Weak and Uncoordinated

The message of this book is probably least agreeable to people who, like me, were skinny and weak as kids or had the wrong body types to be good at sports. Personally, I managed to get through four years of high school without getting a single varsity letter. A minor miracle in that school in those days. I remember spring, ninth grade, when it was time to pick out "club" teams for baseball. A group of us, the unchosen, standing around embarrassed at the end. "Okay, you take those guys. I'll take these guys." Because everyone had to play.

Well, heartening news! In a funny way, people like us have an easier time with this regimen than the gods of our childhood. There are two reasons. First, it's surprisingly hard for serious athletes to come to grips with the fact that they are nowhere near as good as they were at twenty or whatever. They sulk. They drink. They refuse to play. They go to hell. I have a number of athletic pals from childhood who have gone to pieces rather than go out and do athletic stuff at less than optimal levels. I don't know what it's all about; it's not my problem. Or yours, probably. If you were not a sports god as a kid, you don't have to get over yourself. Just doing it is fine. Congratulations.

Second, if you were not a sports god as a kid, there is every reason to anticipate that your Personal Best is still ahead and that you have years and years of getting Younger Every Year. A personal story: I am seventy years old, and I have never skied better in my life. Literally. I was not much of a skier at twenty-eight, to be sure, but now I am a god. Better than, say, 60 percent of the people on a serious mountain on a given day. Do you have any idea what fun that is? To come sweeping down those hills with a turn of speed and a touch of grace at this late stage in the day? I grin for the pleasure of it. Ridiculous old fool? You bet. Shamefully behind people like Emmet who can really ski? You bet. And I love it. Race you to the bottom!

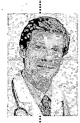

CHAPTER SEVEN

The Biology
of Exercise

Billions of years ago, life on earth divided into two great kingdoms: animals, which move, and plants, which do not. Our ancestors chose movement, and that basic biology hasn't changed since. When you get in shape, when you exercise, when you dance, you are sharing the ancient chemistry of movement with every other animal on the planet.

We can move because we have muscles that contract. Our muscles are sophisticated machines that use oxygen to burn fat or glucose (blood sugar) in millions of tiny engines called mitochondria, which then produce the energy for contraction. It's straightforward internal combustion, just like your car but without a flame. The mitochondria are the key to muscle contraction and to the evolution of movement on earth.

Bacteria developed mitochondria two billion years ago to burn oxygen. Not to produce energy, but to get rid of the oxygen that was just then creeping into the atmosphere and that turned out to be highly toxic stuff, both then and now. It's toxic because it's explosive on a molecular level. That's why fires burn when you add oxygen and why they go out when you remove it. The ability to burn oxygen inside cells is what gives animals the power to move, but free oxygen is dangerous; it burns holes in our DNA, leading to cell death and ultimately to things like heart disease and cancer. Since storing and handling oxygen is such risky business, we have elaborate oxygen detoxification systems that work around the clock to protect us. The antioxidants in the fruits and vegetables we eat soak up the remaining free oxygen (so eat a lot of them) and with all these systems working hard, we get by pretty well. Bacteria didn't have any of this. Instead they used the oxygen to burn sugar in their mitochondria, producing harmless water and carbon dioxide as exhaust.

Five hundred million years ago, bacterial mitochondria somehow moved inside the cells of our primitive ancestors, who harnessed them to their muscles and gave birth to aerobic metabolism. It was access to the unlimited supply of cheap, oxygen-based energy that fueled the explosion of higher life-forms from then on. Bacterial mitochondria make all higher animal life possible, and they live in every muscle cell of every animal on the planet today, including you. All animal motion is fueled by the mitochondria inherited from bacteria—the energy you use to walk in the park, run a marathon, scratch your nose or swim a lap. The DNA in your mitochondria is still bacterial, not human. You inherited it like some ancient, permanent trust fund. Incidentally, plants inherited photosynthesis from algae the same way we stole mitochondria from bacteria, so all life energy on earth today comes from machinery developed by either algae or bacteria.

Pathways to Higher Energy

With that brief look at the last few billion years to put things in perspective, let's talk about getting in shape. Aerobic fitness is all about making more energy in the muscles. That means building more mitochondria and bringing them more fuel and oxygen. Mitochondria can burn either fat or glucose. It's like having a car that can run on either diesel (fat) or gasoline (glucose), depending on your needs: diesel for long-haul road trips, high-octane gasoline for speed and acceleration. Your muscles prefer to burn fat most of the time, because it's a more efficient fuel, but for hard exercise— for speed and power—you burn glucose.

At rest, and with *light* exercise, you burn 95 percent fat and 5 percent glucose. Most fat isn't stored in your muscles; it's stored around your belly and hips and in a few other prime locations. Your body has to bring it to your muscles through your circulation. That's harder than it seems, because your blood is largely water and fat doesn't dissolve in water. Fat has to be carried in special proteins called triglycerides, which your doctor probably mentioned during your last checkup. The trouble with this, from your muscles' perspective, is that your capillaries can handle only a few triglyceride molecules at a time. So each capillary can deliver only a trickle of fat to your mitochondria. With consistent aerobic training, your body builds vast new networks of capillaries to bring more fat to your muscles. Eventually, however, you are delivering as much fat as you possibly can, and if you want to go faster, or harder, you need to start bringing glucose to the mitochondria to use as a second fuel.

With *harder* exercise you keep burning fat in the background, but all the extra energy comes from burning glucose.

Most of the glucose is stored in your muscles ahead of time, but your circulation gets a double workout, first bringing in more glucose and the oxygen necessary to burn it, then carrying away the exhaust, especially the carbon dioxide.

Any way you look at it, circulation is the basic infrastructure of exercise. Steady aerobic exercise, over months and years, produces dramatic improvements in your circulatory system, which is one of the ways exercise saves your life. Exercise stresses your muscles, and they release enough C-6 to trigger C-10. The C-10 released by the adaptive micro-trauma of exercise drives the creation of new mitochondria, the storage of more glucose in the muscle cells and the growth of new capillaries to feed them. Your muscles get hard as you get in shape because they're stuffed full of all the new mitochondria, capillaries and extra glucose. It's a fun image—that newly hardened muscle full of all the stuff you grew by exercising.

The Metabolisms of Hunting and Gathering

Any form of regular, hard aerobic exercise will do the trick, but you can get more mileage out of your exercise if you understand the difference between burning fat and burning glucose. That's the key to really effective aerobic exercise, because different exercise intensities trigger different biological changes throughout your body.

You have two natural aerobic paces, easy and hard, and they depend on two very different muscle metabolisms, which are determined by the fuel you use. Low-intensity, light aerobic exercise burns fat, while high-intensity, hard aerobic exercise burns glucose. It's a critical difference, because these two paces trigger the two distinct metabolisms of foraging and hunting, which are our essential physical rhythms. That's a key point. Those two activities consumed most of our waking hours in nature, and each one called for distinctly different body and brain functions: highly coordinated and specific patterns of thought, mood, energy, digestion, immune function and muscle metabolism. Our bodies and brains geared themselves to our daily environment based largely on our exercise patterns, and that's still how it works today. Never mind that you're walking through the park rather than foraging, or at spin class rather than hunting; light and hard aerobics are still the master control signals for C-6, C-10 and countless other physical and chemical rhythms throughout your body, including your basic brain patterns of behavior and mood. None of this is modern. It's deeply rooted in the mists of evolutionary time, but you can control it by how you exercise.

That's why Chris is going to urge you to buy a heart rate monitor. You need to know how hard you can go burning fat and how hard you can go burning glucose, because that controls health and fitness throughout your body. Your heart rate is the only way to know for sure which metabolism is at work and which signals you're sending. Your heart rate monitor is like the tachometer in a race car: you need to know your rpm to know when to shift gears. Your heart delivers more and more blood to your muscles the faster it pumps, and your muscles can extract more and more fat from that blood until you reach about 65 percent of your peak heart rate. Chris will give you formulas for this in the next chapter, but for an average fifty-year-old, that's a heart rate of 110 beats per minute. If you're sixty-five, it's about 100 beats per minute. That's the number you look for on the dashboard; it's a good, stiff walking pace for most of us, and it's the limit of your first gear in nature.

As soon as you push your body a little harder, you start burning glucose in addition to fat, and you need more oxygen to do this. That means bringing more blood to the muscles, so your heart rate goes up. Any heart rate north of 65 percent means that you're burning glucose and that you've moved into a different metabolism. You've shifted into second gear.

Your body starts drawing on the glucose stored in your muscles, feeding it into your mitochondria to produce the extra energy you need to run and hunt. At some point, however, the glucose metabolism also has an upper limit. You can bring loads of oxygen into the blood and carry away a lot of carbon dioxide, but above a certain level of exertion, the chemicals just can't move between blood and muscle, or within the muscle, fast enough to keep up with the demand. That happens at a heart rate of around 80 percent of maximum. For the fifty-year-old, that's a heart rate of 136 per minute; at sixty-five, it's 124. If you go above your number, your muscles become starved of oxygen and the glucose can't burn all the way down to carbon dioxide. Instead, you build up a sludge called lactate, which is incompletely burned sugar and which shuts down your muscle function after a few seconds of exercise at peak levels (like sprinting the length of a football field). As with the switch from fat to glucose, the switch into "anaerobic" metabolism, where there isn't enough oxygen, has ripple effects throughout your body.

The only way to tell when you reach and cross these thresholds is with a heart rate monitor. You can't do it by how you feel. Even Olympic athletes, training six hours a day for years, can't do it by how they feel. You can certainly get in shape without a heart rate monitor, but you'll waste a fair amount of your time and effort.

Light Aerobic Exercise:
Distance, Not Speed

The concept that exercise intensity is a master signal that regulates chemistry throughout your body and brain is so important that it's worth a closer look, starting with light exercise. Light aerobic exercise is long and slow exercise at an easy pace—up to 65 percent of your peak heart rate. At this level, your muscles burn mostly fat, so it's your most fuel-efficient pace, the one you can keep up all day. It's the pace you once used for foraging and now use for walking miles—for those times when speed doesn't count, but mileage does. You might think it's a waste of time to exercise in this zone, but it's a wonderful pace. This is the metabolic zone where your body and brain heal and grow. It's the zone where steady, low-grade C-10 drives the slow, consistent growth of infrastructure: blood vessels and mitochondria in your muscles; repair and health throughout your body. You become more fit with harder exercise, but you gain more endurance and general healthiness with prolonged light exercise. Do this outdoors with your heart rate monitor and you'll love it. Learn what it's doing for you inside and you'll become an addict.

Let's go for a walk on the beach and talk about this some more. When you first wake in the morning, your body is still asleep and your muscles are in hibernation, running on a trickle of blood and burning fat in the metabolic equivalent of a pilot light. As you stretch and greet the day, the changes begin. Simply opening your eyes activates large parts of your brain, releases adrenaline and increases blood flow to your muscles. Your heart rate rises a few beats as you roll out of bed. You start to move, to walk and shave and shower, and your heart speeds up, pumping out more blood with each stroke. Arteries dilate throughout your legs, forcing oxygen-rich blood deep into the muscle fibers, sending the chemical signals that bring your body to life. Your knees and hips pump their lubricating fluid around, and the stiffness slowly leaves your joints. Have a light breakfast, finish your coffee and head out the door to the beach, where another beautiful day has started.

Sand between your toes, early morning sun coming off the water. Give yourself five minutes of slow, relaxed strolling to warm up, then ease into a good, stiff walk. You could keep this up for miles. And you feel that way for the first twenty minutes of the walk. You're taking it easy, and your muscles are burning fat over a low flame. As you loosen up and start to hit your stride, the fat burns hotter and faster. When you hit about 65 percent of your heart's maximum output, your leg muscles are working at the upper limit of their low aerobic zone. ("Aerobic" means your muscles have all the oxygen they need.) This is as fast as you can go burning fat. It's like diesel: great mileage but low torque. You can go all day, but you can't go fast.

Well, it turns out you don't have to, because you've walked steadily into C-10 territory. Think of growth and repair in terms of a public works project: building an interstate takes time, and new capillaries don't sprout up all at once after the first day at the gym. Your body thinks about it for a while, plans the route and organizes the materials before it starts construction. Your body also doesn't trust you, or, more accurately, it doesn't trust nature. If you fall off track for a little while, even for a distressingly short interval of sloth, construction stops. The real benefits of exercise come with months and years of sustained, steady growth. Short-term gains in fitness are fun but misleading. They depend on surges of C-10—metabolic tricks your body uses to forage during the January thaw, ready to hibernate the moment the cold snap hits again. Months and years of exercise are different. They produce the slow, deep currents of C-10 that sustain the steady engagement of your infrastructure in long-term growth.

This all happens automatically through a carefully choreographed chemical dance within your bloodstream and body. The C-10 pattern of long, slow exercise regulates literally dozens of chemical signals in your body and brain. Names you might recognize, like growth hormone, testosterone, insulin, adrenaline and serotonin; names you don't, like endothelial growth factor, tumor necrosis factor and platelet-derived growth factor. The point is that long, slow exercise builds your muscles, heart and circulation, mobilizes your fat stores and then goes beyond that to let your body heal. Long, slow exercise is the opposite of the chronic inflammation of modern living. It's the tide of youth.

With training, you can easily double the circulatory and mitochondrial capacity you had before you started. Several months of long, slow exercise will turn you into a happy, Zen-like powerhouse of aerobic capacity. Zen-like because your brain does not know you're walking on the treadmill. It thinks you're foraging, and it moves automatically into the chemical state where your mind is engaged but relaxed. Your thinking is clear; your mood is calmer and more alive than it was at rest. Your brain wave patterns on an EEG are similar to meditation states, and for good reason—this is the pace you used in nature when the threat was low.

What's interesting is that the actual pathways of relaxation and focus in your brain become stronger with use. Long-term memory improves with regular exercise, and the risk of Alzheimer's drops. Long hikes and long, easy bike rides are the kinds of low aerobics we prefer, because frankly it's pretty tedious walking slowly on the treadmill for an hour or more. Besides, it makes sense to try to put the mental and physical sides of foraging back together. Rowing an hour to your favorite fishing hole is a wonderful way to start a summer day. Hiking five miles into the forest to bird-watch is perfect foraging, and biking twenty miles on a weekend morning is pure heaven.

Hard Aerobics: Pushing the Herd

Exercising hard enough to push your heart rate above 65 percent calls for a new fuel. You need more power than you can get from fat alone, so your muscles start to burn glucose. This shift into high gear changes your metabolism because harder exercise is the automatic signal that you've started to hunt.

Here's how it works. Animals in nature *never* move out of their low aerobic zone unless they're hunting, being hunted or playing (rehearsal for the first two). Glucose is powerful but expensive fuel. Your body knows that you would *never* move fast enough to burn glucose while foraging. That would be a waste of energy, which is to say that it would be biologically insane. If you're burning glucose, you must be hunting, which triggers a major metabolic shift that affects your muscles, brain, gut, immune system, kidneys, liver, heart and lungs.

Picture this: Prey is in sight. Adrenaline surges, C-6 surges, nonessentials shut down and blood floods your active muscles. You become engaged and alert. You notice more; your step has more bounce. In the lab, with harder exercise, whole new areas of your brain light up on functional MRI scans; you process visual information faster and do calculations more quickly; your attention goes outward, your reflexes sharpen and your salivary flow increases. Back on the beach, this means you're warmed up, fully engaged and ready to run. As you hit your stride, your head comes up, your nostrils flare and your pupils dilate. You feel more alive, clearheaded and younger. Not because of anything conscious, but because you've automatically turned on a whole series of complex control mechanisms by exercising harder.

Your arms swing freely, you breathe more deeply and your legs start to really work. You feel a surge of energy as your heart rate climbs steadily past 65 percent. Welcome to the high aerobic zone. You have just started to burn glucose—your high-octane gasoline equivalent. Not such great mileage, but a lot more power. You keep burning that low level of fat in the background, but all the extra fuel from this point on up is glucose.

All those days of long, slow exercise you did earlier built you a bigger engine. Now, with glucose added, those extra mitochondria and blood vessels are running on rocket fuel. This is the benefit of low aerobic training. It's a trick nature invented so you could catch the antelope, and it's why every endurance athlete in the world does long and slow to build the base fitness for harder aerobics. Every Olympic hopeful, every world record holder, every rider in the Tour de France does it, and so should you. Remember, they are merely chasing gold; you are chasing youth.

And it gets better, because as important as long and slow is, adding hard aerobics makes your body faster and more powerful still. It drives your body to store more glucose right in the muscles, making them ready for sustained, hard exercise.

Nature's perspective on hard aerobic exercise is that you are designed to be an endurance predator, able to work with your buddies to run down antelopes on the savannah. You may not feel much like an endurance predator, but you are. You are designed to be able to circle the antelope herd for hours, running them hard enough to find out which are the weak and old. A person in good shape has enough glucose in his muscles for about two hours of hard exercise. Not full out, but a pretty good effort. Two hours of pushing the herd.

This is also why exercise kicks your brain into high gear. Not to write *War and Peace,* but to eat. Think about tracking hundreds of caribou for hours across the tundra, picking out individuals, assessing their fitness, watching them run, marking and remembering your prey. That's the brain function you turn on with high aerobic exercise. The intense concentration, excitement, physical power, challenge and opportunity of hunting is automatic, it's healthy and it's fun. And the more you hunt, the better your brain gets at this.

Hard aerobics, working up a good sweat, is our favorite exercise rhythm because hunting brings out our youngest and best biology: strong, fast, energetic and optimistic all day long. That's why you should do low aerobic exercise a couple of days a week to build your base, and then go out and play hard on the high-aerobic fields the other days. Tell your body it's springtime.

Anaerobic Exercise: The Lactate Burn

One of the nice things about stepping out of nature is that most of us no longer need to kill to eat or worry about being killed. But when we did, we had an extra gear to call on—ten seconds of raw power for what wildlife biologists call "escape or capture" moments.

You can push the glucose pace all the way up to about 85 percent of your maximum heart rate, where you hit the limit of your high aerobic capacity. That's the fastest pace you can sustain, but for a few seconds you can go faster still. In a burst of youthful enthusiasm at the beach, you can sprint 100 yards to the top of a dune. You double your power output for those last 300 feet. Your heart is putting out 400 percent of its resting capacity, and still you go way beyond its ability to deliver blood and oxygen. You kick in the after-burners for that burst of power, dumping energy into your muscles in a controlled chemical explosion. You have gone anaerobic, your third metabolic gear, the realm beyond oxygen. Sand is flying, your arms are pumping, your heart is pounding, legs burning, you can't keep it up any longer—and suddenly you're standing on top of the dune, winded but fully alive.

That's not aerobic exercise, it's not endurance training and it's not something you should do every day, but it's fun to play with. It's anaerobic exercise, where there's no oxygen in your muscles. It's also your oldest metabolic pathway, dating back to the days when there was no oxygen on earth, before the bacteria invented mitochondria. It's more primitive than aerobic metabolism: less efficient and less biochemically elegant, but far more powerful over short distances and a critical gear to have in the evolutionary transmission. It saved your ancestors' lives, or let them end someone else's, countless times over the past few billion years.

Playing at anaerobic levels is a great way to get in peak shape. It's the ultimate hunting signal. It doesn't do anything for longevity, or probably for overall health, but it's great for vim, vigor and pure fitness. Don't bother with it until you get into pretty good basic shape, then add in interval training a couple of times a week. It's not the key to the rest of your life, but a little bit of escape/capture is important once you're back in predator mode. It's the climax of the hunt, standing victorious on top of the dune.

Make It Happen

Exercise is the friendly trick you play on nature. Your body expects you to walk ten miles a day, with an hour or two of hunting and some sprinting and heavy labor thrown in, but fortunately it's not that smart. You can convince it that spring has come to the savannah with just under an hour a day of exercise. Less than an hour a day to be lean, fit, alert, energetic, healthy and optimistic for decades to come.

Nature is not a treadmill at the gym. It's an ever-changing physical environment, so it should come as no surprise that a variety of different exercises and intensities do more good than a single, unvarying routine. Practically speaking, most people also burn out on any given exercise program over time, so we suggest incorporating a lot of variety over the next thirty years. Nature's rule is simple: *Do something real every day.* Ignore all that talk out there about exercising three or four days a week. Ignore it! Like our national cholesterol guidelines, it's a bare minimum, a desperate plea from the medical profession to a nation of couch potatoes. Remember, your body craves the *daily* chemistry of exercise. Whether the exercise is long, slow and steady (an hour or two of good, hard walking) or shorter and more intense (running, swimming or using the exercise machines at the gym) is a lot less important than the "dailyness" of it, six days a week. So experiment with a variety of different aerobic exercises at the gym, and work hard to find some outdoor sports that you like: biking, kayaking, downhill or cross-country skiing or stiff hiking. Keep your heart rate in the high aerobic zone at the gym and in the low aerobic zone while exercising outside, and you'll get great results. Remember that the whole point is to give your body and brain the sustained signals that tell them to grow younger. It's not important whether you get younger quickly or slowly; you have plenty of time. What *is* important is to keep moving in the right direction.

Showing Up

People don't fall off track because they do the wrong exercises at the gym. They fall off track because they stop going, just for a day or two, and then never go back. I've worked on this with thousands of patients, and it's the *habit and routine* of exercise that lead to success.

And that's not so easy. We are hardwired to eat, to make love and to sit down and rest whenever we can because in nature it was not clear when—or whether—the opportunity would come again. Now, in times of plenty and ease, those instincts are disastrous, but they are never going to go away.

Luckily, you can rewire your brain with structure and routine. Just take that amazing life skill you started building the first day you showed up for kindergarten and turn it to a new purpose. Show up at the gym. Think of it as a great job, which it is. It will change your life, slowly but surely, because once you show up you are virtually certain to do some meaningful exercise. *And even if you don't, you will show up again tomorrow.* That's the key—showing up again tomorrow for the rest of your life.

It makes sense to think of this as a job because once you pass the age of fifty, exercise is no longer optional. You have to exercise or get old. Chris doesn't wake up and think about whether or not to go to the gym every day, any more than he woke up and thought about whether or not to go to work. No matter how he feels, he gets out of bed and he goes. It's easier that way, and he is much, much younger as a result.

The earlier you start, the bigger the payoff, which brings us to the decade or so before retirement—to the challenge of exercising while you're still working at full speed. It may seem exhausting to fit exercise into your crazy work schedule, but that's looking at it backwards. We are not tired at the end of the day because we get too much exercise. We are tired because we do not get *enough* exercise. We are mentally, emotionally and physically drained from being sedentary. Walking through the door exhausted each night is not living; it is merely surviving large stretches of the only life we're likely to have. Besides, study after study shows that the productivity gains at work outweigh the time spent exercising, and that we function better at home—with more satisfaction and on less sleep—when we're fit. If you put any value at all on your quality of life, the time you spend exercising becomes a bargain. (If corporations bothered to look at the science, being in great shape would be a job requirement!) The reality is that your life is so full in these years that you can't afford *not* to exercise. The only real issue is that it's tough to keep up the motivation to exercise when life is crowded with obligations and stress. So rely on structure more than motivation. Carve out the time to exercise, make it "protected time" and guard it fiercely against intrusion.

Getting Started

The jump-in-at-the-deep-end strategy happened to work for Chris, but the risk of injury is relatively high if you're out of shape. Start out by pushing yourself hard enough to sweat, but at a level that matches your current fitness. The worse shape you're in and the older you are, the more important it is to keep each day's exercise well within your limits. This means keeping the intensity low and building up the duration. Remember the chemistry of inflammation? Well, for decades all those C-6 chemicals in your bloodstream have been telling your joints to decay. Arthritis is largely an inflammatory disease of sedentary societies: it's a disease of C-6. So after a few decades of decay your joints are *old*— older than your heart, your arteries, your lungs, your brain, and older than your muscles by decades. If you make this into a contest between your muscles and your joints, your joints will lose. Show up every day, but take it at your own pace as you settle into harness. Finally, no matter how fit you are, check with your doctor before you start any of this, and ask if you need a stress test.

There Are No Limits

Getting into great shape is fun and wonderful if you're healthy, but it's essential if you're not. Even if you're in truly lousy shape now, or if something really bad happens to you down the road, take heart—everyone can do this. I have patients who didn't come to regular exercise until *after* strokes, cancer or heart attacks, but once they did, their lives improved dramatically. Arthritis, strokes, heart attacks, brain tumors, prostate cancer and a host of other woes may put limits on what *kind* of exercise you do, but none of them can stop you.

I walk to work through New York City's Central Park (one of the world's great commutes), and for at least a decade I've watched an old guy running there. He must have had a major stroke, because he has the strangest, floppiest gait I've ever seen. Apparently, he can only really run with the good half of his body and just throws the other half forward in an act of faith with each step. The stroke probably affected his temperature regulation as well, because he never wears a shirt. But he's out there—skinny old chest, shirt off in 20-degree snowstorms, looking prehistoric and, as far as I can tell, living the hell out of his life. There is something enormously appealing about seeing this guy appear out of a snowstorm, half naked, with his queer, lopsided gait, but so *alive*. It doesn't matter who he is, he's facing a lot more than you, Chris or me, and he is triumphant because he shows up day after day, year after year. Remember this guy when you think you can't exercise. He had a stroke and can barely walk, so he *really* can't exercise. But he does, and I bet he loves it. You will, too.

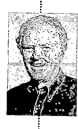

CHAPTER EIGHT

The Heart of the Matter: Aerobics

Think of that . . . we can burn either diesel or gasoline, at a whim, whenever we want. That's amazing. There isn't a car on the road that can do that. And we can burn stuff without using oxygen at all. A miracle. May we respectfully suggest that the least you can do to show your appreciation for this marvelous machine is to keep it in something like working order? And not just out of gratitude. If you let it get mucked up with blacky carbon and gummy sludge, it will blow up. And kill you dead. Well, maybe not dead, but open-heart surgery. Did Harry have a chance to talk about open-heart surgery? I didn't think so. Consider it for a minute, to strengthen your appetite for this slightly pedestrian chapter. Open-heart surgery is hugely popular these days, apparently because so many guys prefer it to reading about aerobics and working out.

The surgery's not really that tricky anymore. All the surgeons have to do is cut open your chest with a knife, then crack your sternum like the shell of a lobster with a huge pair of shears. Snip, snip, snip. And then the team—don't worry, they've done this a thousand times—cranks the bones back so the doc can reach in and . . . Hey, you don't want to hear about open-heart surgery, do you? You think it's scary and disgusting. Fine. Some heart patients say it's not as bad as it sounds but that it's, well, intrusive. Exercise is intrusive, too . . . takes up almost an hour a day, which is a lot. You can skip it if you like, along with this chapter. But you may eventually have to learn that skin-the-lobster trick. My preference? I'd read a little further.

Long-Term Goals

Let's assume you feel queasy about open-heart surgery. What do you do? Endurance exercise, of course. Send those critical signals to your cells. And the best way to do that is to set long-term goals and get to work on them. The most important one is this: A year from now, you should be able to do long and slow aerobics (that's breathing hard but still able to talk; it's 60–65 percent of your maximum heart rate) for, say, three hours without getting exhausted. You should be able to do that in your sixties, seventies and eighties . . . and a variation of it in your nineties. That's an all-morning bike ride or a hike at a firm pace. You should do something like that, oh, once a month. Two hours is okay some months, but three is better; make it a real outing, a real commitment. Make it a focus of your training, while reminding yourself that this is what it's all about. If you can get to that level of fitness, and stay there, life will be good and you can probably keep the lobsterman at bay. But we think you should do more. You should certainly add strength training, discussed in Chapters Ten and Eleven, because that addresses a whole different set of issues. You should also do aerobics at higher levels so that you can get other fuel systems involved. But remember John on the beach down there in Florida. He never got beyond long and slow, and he's one of our heroes.

Let's keep going. For a second endurance goal, you should be able to do high-endurance aerobics for an hour (that's a serious clip where you can no longer talk, other than a few panted words; it's 70–85 percent of your maximum heart rate). If you can maintain this pace for two hours, that's wonderful. But watch it, you may be turning into an athlete. An hour at this clip is a lot, and it's not easy. Reach that goal and you'll be in super shape.

Finally and least urgently, you should be able to do real hell-for-leather sprints or some other flat-out activity at anaerobic levels (that's everything you've got until you *have* to stop) for a minute or two. This is the least important goal, but it's worth considering. As you know, it uses a different fuel and combustion system (the super-turbo, no-oxygen gear that works so well and makes such a mess afterwards), and it's nice to have all three systems in working order. It's also nice to know that your ancient "fight or flight" mechanism is there if you need it. I like to ring this bell at least once a week, but tastes vary.

The Utter Necessity of Getting a Heart Monitor

Now that you have some goals, how do you get there? The first step is an odd one. You buy a heart monitor. If you haven't been in training for a while, all those references to "percent of your maximum heart rate" in the last section may strike you as arcane and not very useful. Who in the world knows his maximum heart rate or the percentage he's using? The answer is, everyone who is even borderline serious about endurance training. All modern endurance athletes know precisely what level they're working out at, *all the time,* and you should, too. Modern training is always cast in terms of going at different levels of intensity (different percentages of maximum heart rate) for different periods of time and for different purposes. The heart monitor is the tool that lets you build and maintain a strong aerobic base. It works better than anything else you can afford, and it makes the whole business of endurance training a lot more interesting.

A heart monitor is a simple device that tells you how many times a minute your heart beats. That's it. You can get one that analyzes your spit and remembers your mother's maiden name, but you don't need all that. The simplest and cheapest model is fine. But you can't do without one; a heart monitor is as important to your training as a decent pair of sneakers.

People resist this advice like crazy. Maybe because it's new. Or a little bit creepy. You *do* have to put this black strap under your already embarrassing tits, like an aging S&M nut. And it *is* a computer . . . a few folks still resist that. It gets in the way of your endless lying about how hard you work out, too, which is unpleasant. You may find other reasons for not doing it. Well, fine! It's your miserable body. But you should know this: *Every single soul who cares about training swears by the heart monitor.* Every single one, from Lance Armstrong right down to me. It is the device that defines the terms for everyone's workouts. Including yours.

A heart monitor is a two-piece gizmo: one piece is like a wristwatch and the other a band you put around your chest.

Simplest thing in the world. The band picks up your heartbeat and radios the news to the watch. Tells you how many
beats per minute (bpm), instantaneously and constantly. Not
bad for seventy bucks, which is what the cheapest of these
gadgets goes for in discount places.

You can read the directions, if you're the type, or you can
just be a guy, strap it on and work out for a couple of days.
See what you see. Figure out your theoretical maximum heart
rate using this simple formula: 220 minus your age. That
gives a rough maximum heart rate number. Pretty soon, you'll
want something more accurate, but this is fine for now. Then
just go through your normal workout and look down once in
a while; see what percentage of your max you're working at.
Do not try to go to your theoretical max until you're in really
great shape, if ever.

At some fairly early point, you might also want to know
your resting heart rate. There are hip communities where

Figuring Out Your Target Heart Rate

L et's take some baby steps, because this is important. First,
subtract your age from 220. If you're sixty, you'll get 160.
That's your theoretical max. Now take 60 percent of that. (You
don't need a pencil and paper: 60 percent of 100 is 60. Okay?
And 60 percent of 60 is 36. Add 'em up. Sixty percent of your
max is 96. There you go. Now do it for 70 percent. Do it for 80
and 90 percent, too. Memorize those numbers. Or do the math
again in your head, you clever fellow. Fight Alzheimer's.) The
three paces, as you should know by now, are long and slow
(60–65 percent of max), high endurance (70–85 percent of max)
and anaerobic (85–100 percent of max). Know your personal
beats-per-minute for those three ranges.

people talk about their resting heart rate at cocktail parties; you might as well be ready. Your resting heart rate is a vague index of the kind of shape you're in. More importantly, *changes* in your resting heart rate are a pretty good indicator of your own relative condition from day to day. The way you get it is like this: Put the gadget on the bedside table when you go to bed. When you wake up the next morning, put on the strap and put the watch on your pillow where you can see it. Go back to sleep. Almost. When you're drowsy and can barely open your eyes, sneak a peek at the monitor. What does it say? Is it around 50 . . . 60 . . . 70? Good. That's your resting heart rate. Tell everyone about it. Over time, as you get in better shape, your resting heart rate should go down some. And if you wake up some morning and it's abnormally high, that may be a sign that you're coming down with a cold. Or you're hungover. Or you're overtraining. Or your heart is going to stop later in the day (just kidding). If your resting heart rate is high, back off on the intensity of your workouts for a while, until your resting heart rate comes back down.

Harry thinks that knowing your resting heart rate is the cat's whiskers. If you agree, you'll want to check it every morning without the monitor. (We're weird, but we're not going to suggest you keep your heart monitor as a bedside companion for the rest of your life.) Just check it the old-fashioned way—with a finger poked in to find your pulse, just behind your Adam's apple. Keep your eye on a second hand someplace, and start counting. That system is too slow and cumbersome to use on the road or on your bike, but it's fine for this once-a-day test.

This next bit is much more important. Once you're in decent shape, you'll want to figure out your *real* maximum heart rate, which is probably higher than the one you get with the simple formula. If you use the wrong max, all the per-centages—and all of our excellent advice—become useless.

The way to get your real max is to work out pretty damn hard. Once you're in great shape, crank it up until you're doing, say, 90 percent of your theoretical max. How do you feel? Do you have another 10 percent in you before you fall on your face? Try it out. Sniff around your theoretical max, if you feel pretty good. Go beyond it, if you can. Remember, your max is the real-world peak—the pace you can maintain for only sixty seconds or so, going flat out. Don't try to get to your actual max unless you're in fabulous shape (and you've had that physical we told you to get), but get up into the neighborhood and assume that that's 90 or 95 percent of your actual max. Recalculate your numbers, based on the new assumption. It's worth going through all this. My theoretical max, for example, is 150. My actual max is 170. That's a huge difference, and if I were not aware of it, my workouts would get all messed up.

Another route to finding your real max is during a stress test. That should be easy, but, I must tell you, most stress test administrators are not into this. It takes longer, and they don't care what your real max is. So you have to push pretty hard and insist that you want to stay on the treadmill as long as you *possibly* can. But it is nice to reach for your max with a heart doc standing right there . . . just in case you hit it a lit-tle *too* hard.

Recovery Rate

W/ant another number you can boast about? Try your recovery rate—the speed with which your heart rate drops in the sixty seconds after you've gone from peak exertion to a walk. This is the best, most readily available indicator of your aerobic fitness. Let's say you're thrashing along on your stationary bike at 130 beats per minute, which is, maybe, 80 percent of your max. Now just pedal easily and watch both the monitor and the second hand on a watch. The instant your heart rate drops one beat (be sure to wait for it to go down one tick before you start timing; it often goes up when you first slow down), start timing. See how many beats per minute your heart rate drops in sixty seconds. Anything over 20 bpm is satisfactory, more is better. If it drops less than 20, you need a lot more work on your aerobic base. If your recovery rate goes to 30 or 40, tell absolutely everyone you know. It will bore them stupid. The day it hits 50, please call Harry and tell him. I would like to know, too, but I will probably be busy that day.

A One-Hour Hike in the Mountains

And now for a live demonstration of the heart monitor at work . . . it may give you a better idea of how it functions and why it's worth fooling with. I wrote part of this book last winter, during a work/ski vacation in Aspen, where we lived for a while. Most mornings I'd work out for an hour or so before sitting down to the computer. Here's one of those workouts.

It's the fourth day of our stay. I'm used to the altitude, but I'm still on New York time so I'm up at five. It's dark out, even after breakfast, but I can see that it snowed several inches last night. I dress warmly in layers, grab the dog and drive to the bottom of the Smuggler Mine Trail. Aengus, the Weimaraner, is ten years old, but he's doing 360s in the snow while I lace up my boots. He loves this stuff, and so do I. Old boys at play.

Smuggler is a steep Jeep trail that rises from about 7,800 feet to some 9,000 feet, all of it affording stunning views of the little town and the ski mountains. I can do the round trip in about an hour in heavy boots in the snow. Local kids probably do it in half that time. At the bottom, I look at my watch and my heart monitor. Resting heart rate: 65. That's great.

I know the climb well and use the monitor to regulate my pace. Warm up at 100–105 bpm (60 percent of my personal maximum heart rate) for the first five minutes. Then up to about 120 bpm (70 percent) for another five minutes. I feel as if I'm walking pretty hard, so I look down at the monitor to check. Oops: 112. I take a deep breath and pick up the cadence. It's amazing how often you *think* you're working out at a certain level but are actually doing less. Gotta have that heart monitor. A third of the way up, I want to get into the mid-130s (high endurance, or 70–85 percent) for ten or fifteen minutes as the road gets steeper and the air a little thinner. There's a telephone pole two-thirds of the way up . . . a steep patch. I want to be at 140 (82 percent) when I get there. I speed up slightly and hit 140 just at the pole. Good.

Good views, too. I can see the Sno-cats working on a race course on the big mountain. Buses and cars full of workmen, coming in from down valley. Breathtaking scenery all around. This is high-endurance aerobics at the high end.

Okay, a little steeper here, and I hold the cadence . . . maybe lengthen the stride a bit and get into the upper 140s. My personal maximum heart rate is 170, so 145 is about 85 percent, a serious effort. I want to have an anaerobic rush at the end . . . get up into the low 150s, or 90 percent for me. If you're in shape, you're not going to blow a head valve at 90 percent, even at altitude, but it does clear your pipes.

We're rounding the last, long switchback. I'm huffing and my glasses are steamed. Tip back my fur hat . . . try to cool down a little.

Still in the mid-140s, I push a bit and break into a very slow jog . . . careful on the snow and ice. Pounding along now, pulling like a train, around the last turn and up to the little platform at the top. Bingo! Okay, it took twenty-eight minutes, which is good for me with this footing. And, more important, my heart rate is peaking at 157 bpm, or about 92 percent. Excellent. I can only do a few minutes at this anaerobic level, but that's fine. I have given myself a serious aerobic workout—tougher than I would have managed without a heart monitor—and amused myself, too. That counts.

Now recovery. I immediately check my stopwatch and the monitor and time myself for sixty seconds from the first instant my pulse starts to go down from 157. Time! Good. It has dropped to 120, or 37 bpm, in sixty seconds. That's terrific. A strong assurance that I'm in pretty good aerobic shape. I may ski into a tree this afternoon, but I probably won't have a heart attack. No guarantees—the heart's a joker—but probably not. I head down the hill at a serious clip, but I can barely hold my heart rate at 60 percent of max. If the footing weren't so slippery, I'd run to keep it a little higher, but I don't want to break my neck. Very important not to bust anything. A couple of times we stop because Aengus has ice stuck between his paws; he still gets to the car ahead of me. We've been gone an hour. Like endurance predators everywhere, we stop to pick up the local paper, get another cup of coffee and head home. No one else is awake yet; we have stolen a march on the day. And beaten back the tide. All with the help of a little gadget that costs less than seventy bucks.

A Basic Program of Aerobics

Okay, back to basics. We keep protesting that this is not an exercise book, and that's true, but it's going to look an awful lot like one for the next few pages. The reason is that many of Harry's patients and other pals of ours ask for a simple exercise program to get them through the first weeks and months of working out. So we have put together a one-size-fits-all, three-level regimen. Remember, of course, that one size does *not* fit all in this business, so you'll have to tune it to suit yourself. For example, some people—perhaps many—will spend a long time at Levels One and Two, regardless of how fit they get. We think that everyone should add weight training at some point—that's Level Two—but once you've done that, you can stay at the long-and-slow level forever, if you prefer, even though we think there's a lot to be said for getting into high-endurance and anaerobic exercise. Your choice. Our only caveat is this: Don't kid yourself. Start where you should start and stay there until you're really ready to move on. Consistency trumps intensity every time.

If you're a serious athlete, you may be off our exercise charts from the beginning. That's fine. Make your own way with your own trainer or with one of the books on serious endurance training referred to in the Authors' Notes. But there's one thing that does apply to you, no matter how fit you are, and that is the *mix* of different kinds of exercise we're recommending (eventually aerobic exercise at different levels four days a week and at least two days a week of strength training). That mix is as important to you as to anyone else; maybe more so. If you're one of the surprising number of very fit men who train only for a particular sport, your body will get less and less tolerant of that kind of concentration with the passing of years. The systems and muscle groups that you're ignoring will atrophy and raise hell with the rest of your body.

This is all summarized in our exercise program in the Appendix, but it may help to walk you through it in some detail. First, whether you're pretty fit or in god-awful shape, put on your workout duds and your heart monitor, go to the gym or out on the road *and warm up*! Temperamentally, I am not the warm-up type, but even I have become a true believer. At my age, I can feel the difference. And whether it's happened to you or not, sometime in your fifties or sixties you'll realize that it takes much longer for your blood to start moving and for your muscles and joints to warm up. I need five minutes these days and sometimes ten. Feel your own way, but don't skimp just because you're in a hurry or feeling great. Even $10 million athletes are forced to warm up so they won't get hurt. The same applies to you.

Here's another thing: A good warm-up is *the* great antidote to injury, and the risk of getting hurt is different as you get older. First, it's easier to get hurt. Second, it's harder to recover. So, warm up.

After the warm-up, slowly increase the intensity of your biking or jogging or whatever you're doing, and get your heart rate up to 60–65 percent of your max and level off. Keep it up for ten or fifteen or twenty minutes that first day, whatever is comfortable. Cool down for a few minutes. Maybe do some stretches. Go home. You have just started the sacred process of building your aerobic base . . . adding a few mitochondria, stringing a few new capillaries, sending some new signals to your whole body. Maybe giving yourself a squirt of C-10. Nice work. Very nice work.

Next day, do the same thing. If the first day knocked you sideways, do less. If you feel pretty good, do more. Keep inching along at the long-and-slow level—with your heart rate at 60–65 percent of max—for all of the first week and maybe for much longer. Your goal is to go long and slow for forty-five minutes without getting wrecked. (Ultimately, of course, you want to be able to do two or three hours of this.) If, at the end of the first week or the second or the third, you still cannot go at 60–65 percent for forty-five minutes, that's fine; just keep on keeping on. It's the very best thing you can do. There's no rush. Building your aerobic base is the most important aspect of this regimen.

One of the tip-offs that you are *not* ready to move on is something you can only get from your heart monitor. If you're tooling along on your treadmill or your bike at 65 percent of your max and your heart rate suddenly spikes up ten or fifteen points, even though you're not working any harder, you've reached your temporary wall for the day. Slow down or, more likely, quit. Resume long and slow the next day.

I'm talking about a spike, not a "drift" upward of five or six beats a minute. Everyone experiences some upward drift after he's been working out for a while, regardless of the shape he's in. Just this morning, I was having an extended long-and-slow day—an easy all-morning bike ride at 60–65 percent of my max. Toward the end, I was biking at about the same clip but my heart rate had gone up to 70 percent. That's drift, not a spike. No reason to slow down or stop. But if it goes to 75–80 percent of max, slow down, or quit and come back tomorrow. If you're just beginning to work out after a long layoff, you may hit that wall in ten minutes, not two hours. No problem.

At some point, you should add weights to take you to Level Two. We talk about that in Chapters Ten and Eleven, but I mention it here so you can have a complete sense of the program. Read the chapters on strength training before you start, but add weights at some point. Earlier is better.

Eventually, a workout should last forty-five minutes to an hour, including the warm-up and cooldown. That's true of both aerobic and strength training. You can add more time eventually, but forty-five minutes to an hour, six days a week, is plenty. We are not trying to turn ourselves into athletes here; we are trying to live the good life.

You Are an Endurance Predator: Act like One

Once you can do forty-five minutes of long and slow, it's time to mix in some high-endurance aerobics. That's the next level, the one at which you get to 70–85 percent of your max. It's not absolutely essential that you get to that level, but it's a good idea. First, because you use a whole different fuel system, and it's sensible to keep all your systems working. Second, you get a great high from all the yummy C-10, which high-endurance exercise generates in massive doses.

You might eventually decide that high endurance is not to your taste, but give it a try. Take a spin with that excellent glucose-burning system; see if you like it. No sense having it, really, if you're not going to use it. And, as Harry points out, you were built to operate at these levels. You may not look it these days, but you were. Think of it . . . chubby, old fellows like us, thundering along with our tongues out, running down an eland with our buddies for an hour or two. Running down the tasty wildebeest. Being among the first to reach the carcass. Sounds odd, but you're the man. Give it a shot; it's in your blood.

A high-endurance day should go something like this. Warm up, of course; that never changes. Then up to 60–65 percent of your max for five or ten minutes. Then crank it up to 70–75 percent and hold at that level for five or ten minutes. Feel your way. That's intense enough for your high-endurance work in the early stages and maybe forever. Then back down for recovery at 60–65 percent. Over time, be sure to amuse yourself with variations. Make it hard enough to be interesting, but not so hard that you're knocked out. Eventually, you should be able to hold at 70–75 percent for twenty minutes without much strain. After a while, as you know, you should be able to hold it at 70–85 percent of max for an hour or two without flying apart.

If you have trouble getting up to the 70–85 percent level, think about aerobics classes of some kind. I often find it hard to make myself go to high endurance all alone, even though I know it's great for me and that it will feel good. I feel a terrible temptation to dog along at 60–65 percent. But in spinning class I *always* get up in the high-endurance range; indeed, that's what spinning is all about. Other types of classes do the same thing.

Or consider a demanding bike ride or hike, like the one I described taking in Colorado. Most of us don't have a serious hiking opportunity in the backyard, but there are lots of ways to skin the high-endurance cat, and not all of them involve sucking in someone else's exhaust and being yelled at in the gym.

Fight or Flight: Dodging Traffic

The final aerobic stage—adding some real sprints or doing intervals to go to the anaerobic level (85–100 percent of your max)—is completely optional, though pretty good fun if you're in shape. You can't get that special endorphin rush any other way. Or the pleasant knowledge that you won't necessarily be dead meat if you get the ancient "fight or flight" call some dark and stormy night. Going anaerobic is not to be undertaken lightly or unadvisedly, however. It's barely mentioned in our exercise program, because a lot of people of a certain age shouldn't go there. If you do decide to go for it, wait until you're in really good shape and be sure to check with your doctor first. People do die of this stuff.

Okay, the way you get there is this. You go for it. Which probably means doing something along these lines. First, as ever, you warm up. Maybe a little longer than usual, so you won't be as likely to hurt yourself when you really hit it. Then go to, say, 75 percent of your max. On an anaerobic (or "sprint" or "intervals") day, 75 percent is going to be the base you go back to for rest. After ten minutes or so at 75 percent, crank it up to 80–85 percent for a five- or six-minute stretch. Drop back to recovery level (75 percent) for a couple of minutes, then hit it with everything you've got for two minutes. Maybe only one. The object is to get to 85–90 percent of your max at this stage. Now relax and rest at, say, 75 percent of your max for two minutes. Then hit it again, for one minute, as hard as you can. You should be up in the 90th percentile now. Relax for sixty seconds and hit it again. These are "intervals," designed to get your heart rate way up there. You should definitely be in the 90s by this time. You may or may not do a third or fourth interval, but pretty soon it's going to be time for a longer rest, first at 75 percent and then at lower levels. Do one last sprint, if you like, then wind down to 65 percent. Keep working out at low levels until your heart rate drops below 60 percent. Nice work. You're done.

That's our introduction to aerobic exercise. Use our program in the Appendix to get started, then find your own way. Do some kind of aerobic exercise four days a week forever. You'll get to love it, no kidding.

Powder Rules Apply

After soldiering through all this virtuous stuff, you may be thinking, "Is this struggle really worth it?" Well, yes, it really is. You'll feel better *all* the time, and once every so often you'll feel absolutely great. What follows is another payoff story. It should perhaps come after the strength chapters because it involves strength training, too, but you've been through a lot; let's go play in the snow for a few minutes.

One night, toward the end of the Aspen work/ski vacation I mentioned, we had the dump of the year—almost three feet of new snow. The next morning, the ski patrol ran up the EPIC flag at Highlands, which doesn't happen often, and the powder hounds were out in force, calling to one another as they flew down the hills. The powder hounds are the kids who can actually ski this stuff. They live in crummy hotels and tend the bars, park the cars and put up the drywall, just so they can be here on days like this.

They were first in line, and when they got to the top, they headed for the steepest places and went flying down. By long tradition, they yodeled and whooped as they turned, again and again, in the waist-high snow for the sheer joy of the thing. The tourists and the grown-ups, starting their breakfasts down in the town, heard them through the walls and felt a little uneasy. The young waiters who took their orders didn't care much about them that morning, because they heard the whooping, too, and their hearts were in the hills.

I was with Hilary's pal Lois, because Hilary hasn't been able to ski this stuff ever since she broke her neck (not doing exercise!) seven years ago. She's fine, but she can't do this. Lois, forty-four, has an excellent job, an excellent husband and two fine children, but not that morning. That morning, it was his turn to stay home with the kids, and, for her, "Powder

Rules Apply." That's the sign they put up in shop windows when they lock the door and head for the mountain. All bets are off, and appointments will not be kept. Ecstasy trumps care.

Lois learned to ski in the east, and she and Tom moved out here to do it more. She is wonderful company, a total yoga nut, and she is way strong. Which matters a lot. That's one of the dirty little secrets about skiing that the instructors and ski magazines never mention. Skiing is a strength sport. Aerobics and strength. The stronger and fitter you are, the more fun you have. They don't want you to know that, but it's true. There's technique and there's balance. But, time and again, strength and fitness are what make it possible. Especially in powder.

Everyone knows that powder skiing is supposed to be great fun, but frankly most people can't do it for squat. They fall all the time, and it takes forever for them to get up because there's no bottom to push off from. They get scared and sit back on their skis. Fall some more. Their thighs burn. They go home and don't come out again until the snow is packed down. Lois and I were among the first in line. Maybe her kids had breakfast, maybe not. But the EPIC flag was flying and we were *out there*.

Up top, it was blue and clear and the thick-laden trees were sparkling. One of those Rocky Mountain miracles you sometimes get. We should have warmed up on an easier trail, but that would have been a waste. The point of a dump is the steeps and deeps. We hustled over to Northstar . . . big, easy turns in deep powder on the upper part, big, steep turns down below. A couple of skiers had been there before us, but every turn was in virgin snow. Everything is slow motion when you get this right. You're dancing. Very, very slowly, then very, very fast. You feel the swoosh, and the snow flies up over your head. A "face shot," they call it. In the

Bugaboos in the Canadian Rockies, they wear snorkels, sometimes, to breathe. Not here, but it's deep and the snow is incredibly light.

We were in the steeps. There are always moguls on this pitch, but that day they were deep under the snow, like bears asleep under the drifts. We pointed our skis straight down the steepest pitch, dancing around the bears. The gravity pulled us down, the snow held us up. And we danced in between. Lois and I were flying, side by side. We grinned, and we whooped. All the way down. Down the steep, open hill, down through the huge trees in The Glades. Up and across to the Ridge of Bell and into the steeps again.

We did every double black on the hill. Every place it was deep until it was all packed out. We raced back up and swung back down. Half the time we were panting to get our breath at the end of a run. Some places, in the trees where the snow was really ridiculous, we struggled. Great skiers can do this with the same technique as trail skiing, but I needed to get back on my quads so I could steer the skis, wiggle, wiggle, wiggle. By mid-morning, we were soaked in sweat and felt lovely. And we just kept going. Not in pain, I am thrilled to report. My old quads did not hurt, and they would have hurt like crazy ten years ago. Or twenty years ago. I could not have done this then. Even Lois's quads hurt. Quite a bit! I love it. Yoga's great, but there's no substitute for the stinky aerobics and the weights if you're going to do this stuff.

Around two, we were cooked. We had been at it for almost five hours, with pit stops and a quick bite. We got beers and lolled for a while at the bottom, with the other kids. Lois and I were exhausted but delighted with ourselves and with our day. We nattered like children about this run and that. We boasted and took turns praising each other. We thought we were wonderful. We sure *felt* wonderful. Then I went home to bed. Slept for three hours.

When I woke up, it was dark. I would not have needed that sleep forty years ago, but that's okay. That morning, when they flew the EPIC flag at Highlands, I was in my seventieth year. And I was a powder hound in the hills. And I danced and I whooped as I turned. For the sheer joy of my life. And perhaps I was heard in the town . . . where the grown-ups were ordering breakfast.

The Kedging Trick

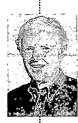

ook, it is not easy to keep doing exercise six days a week, year in and year out, for the rest of your life. You may falter. You may start skipping whole weeks. You may say the hell with it. We recognize, Harry and I, that you may need a little special motivation, three or four times a year, to keep yourself going. We suggest that you familiarize yourself with the notion of "kedging." Never heard of it? Well, it goes like this.

Sailing ships, becalmed and threatened, sometimes had to resort to kedging to get out of trouble. The captain would have a light anchor (a kedge) loaded into a longboat and rowed half a mile or so away. The longboat crew would set the anchor, and everyone back on the big boat would pull like demons on the line, literally hauling the ship to the anchor. Then they'd do it again, until they got where they had to go. Sounds like a lot of work, but maybe worth it if it's the only way to overcome a

tide that's pulling you onto a lee shore or to get under the desperately needed protection of coastal batteries.

So . . . kedging: climbing out of the ordinary, setting a
desperate goal and working like crazy to get there. To save
yourself.

It is our view, Harry's and mine, that you have to do a little kedging now and then to keep yourself motivated. Figure
out your own technique, but what we have in mind is stuff
like booking an adventure trip—skiing, hiking or whatever
—that's beyond your ability and training hard for months to
get in shape to handle it. Then doing it right. Or buying a
piece of gear that's way too good for you and working into
it. Book yourself into a killer spa and do their regimen. Or
take up some entirely new sport or activity, like squash or
yoga, and get good enough at it to know whether you want to
keep it in your life. Sounds like a lot of trouble, but it's fun,
too, and it works. And remember, your life is going to be
very long. You need tricks to keep yourself interested.

The Serotta Solution

When I turned fifty, a long time ago, my kids and some
pals got together and bought me a sensational racing
bike. I hadn't been biking or doing much of anything else for
a while, and they thought that was too bad. They turned to a
man named Ben Serotta for help. At the birthday party, a
cheerful black-tie event, my son Tim rolled out this amazing
blue-and-yellow creation to the oohs of the crowd. I still
remember one line of his speech: "If Ben Serotta had gone
into politics and become a governor, his would have been a
happy and a prosperous people. Luckily, he decided to make
bicycles instead . . ." And so on. Nice night.

It was a serious racing bike and much too short-framed and tender for my modest skills. But it was so damn beautiful —there are few things better-looking on earth than a classic, steel bicycle—that I just couldn't stay off it. I got into biking, big time, and have never looked back. It is at the heart of my exercise life. I've gotten other bikes from time to time, but I still ride the Serotta sometimes, because I'm so grateful to it for getting me back into the sport. A surprising number of men my age are still biking hard, and a surprising number of them spend astonishing amounts on carbon fiber or titanium Treks, Lite-Speeds, Sevens and Lord-knows-whats. Harry has a pal with a barn full of them.

I gather that Ben Serotta is a real star now, and he may not have time, but I mean to call him and see if he wants to give it another shot. It is an interesting assignment: a bike to satisfy a semi-serious seventy-year-old who means to bike pretty steadily, in sickness and in health, for the next quarter of a century. Serotta must be getting on himself these days, but he may want to help design a superlight anchor to kedge me into old age.

Pulling to Paradise

Harry says no one rows anymore, except a handful of people who went to a handful of eastern colleges, so it's dumb or, worse, *elitist* to put my Whitehall in the book, but I don't care. Rowing is not elitist. Decent men have been rowing for pleasure since the dawn of history. It is one of the blessings of humanity. What a genius that first guy was who jumped on a log and paddled across a river, while his enemies stood dumbfounded on the shore. And how about the man who figured out how to sit backwards and row? Or the excellent creature who invented the sliding seat and outriggers, so he could row with his legs as well as his arms? Going about in pulling boats is deep in our blood, and the luckiest of us still do it. I do not say that the man who lives on the water and knows nothing but the inflatable, the Cigarette boat or the diesel knows nothing of the sea. But he doesn't know much.

I have wanted a Whitehall skiff with a sliding seat and outriggers for as long as I can remember. Something to row in heavier weather and open water. When Harry and I sold this book, I had already written the chapter on economy, so I did not squander the advance. But I did buy an overcoat of a curious design, which I had wanted since I was sixteen. And an incredibly beautiful blue pulling boat, made by the good people of Little River Marine, which I named *Yeats* after the poet. She has a lovely wineglass stern and hatchet-shaped oars that are nine feet long and lighter than ski poles. And she pulls like a train . . . one of the nicest motions in the water I have ever felt.

There is no better exercise in the world than rowing a single scull or a Whitehall or any other good pulling boat. It's aerobic, of course, but it exercises your whole body while it immerses you in a rhythm and takes you to places that are good for your soul. Consider yesterday. It was an unusually mild and sunny Thanksgiving, and I rowed all the way from Sag Harbor, Long Island, over to Shelter Island and back, a sweet, three-hour pull. There were no other boats. My pulse was a steady 60–65 percent most of the time, so I was adding hundreds of those pesky mitochondria and miles of capillaries to my aerobic base, but I wasn't thinking about that. I was thinking about the swans beside me, at eye level, and the slap and whir of their huge wings as they rose off the water. About the seal who followed me for a little ways, curious as a dog.

About the magic inlets in the tall marsh grass into which I pulled and sat, invisible, for a while. About the deep, steady rhythm of the rowing and the sweet glide of the boat through the water. And about the good, solid miracle of being younger *this year,* on Thanksgiving Day, on the water, in *Yeats.* For which I was duly grateful. A boat like this is the perfect kedge to pull yourself into . . . well, into eternity, really.

The General Rule of Gear

There is one black-letter rule that you should know and act upon as you get older: Men who are *out there* in their fifties, sixties and beyond—skiing down the shoots, biking in the hills, rowing over the horizon—deserve the best equipment that money can buy. This advice does not quite rise to the dignity of Harry's Rules, but it makes fine sense. It is not so easy, after all, to bike a hundred miles a day when you're in your sixties, to windsurf in high wind in your fifties, to ski the deep powder in your seventies. Come to think of it, it's not *that* easy just to get out of bed in the morning and train, six days a week. So, if you're doing it, you deserve decent gear. Skimp on washing machines and junk like that. Buy good gear.

If you're one of those conservative old boys who pride themselves on using ancient stuff until it falls apart after much mending, get over it. You cannot *fix* stuff to match modern gear. Gear has gotten so much better, in almost every sport, in the last twenty years that you cannot touch it with your old junk. Parabolic skis, for example, have absolutely revolutionized the sport. Made it radically easier to be an intermediate and quite a lot easier to be an expert. Your 1975 Heads were hot when you bought them, but now they're about as hot as the Stem Christie. They don't make them anymore, either, and it's a good thing.

Same with bikes. I love my old Serotta, but it is not in the same league with the new bikes. The gearing is different. The material of the frame is different. The brakes. Everything. And while there is still room in the decent heart for steel (especially if you can afford the elegant Richard Sachs), most steel bikes cannot compare with composites or titanium for a great ride. And peppy? These new bikes practically rear up and whinny when you put your foot down.

Rowing, too. If it's been a while, just wait until you try out those hatchet-shaped, carbon-fiber oars: they are a miracle of effectiveness. To say nothing of a modern, carbon-fiber single scull or a new Whitehall skiff like *Yeats*. Conventional Whitehalls with fixed seats and wooden oars just aren't in it. I own one and I know. Tennis rackets? Same thing. And hiking boots. So give yourself a break and get some decent gear. Buying *Yeats* cracked our budget like an egg, but it's one of the best things I've ever done.

I have had a hellish time with Harry on this subject, because he's so conservative. He was a serious biker as a kid and has a bike on which he literally biked across the country twenty-five years ago. Today, in my modest opinion, it is a lovable piece of junk. But will Harry pitch it and get something good? No! He has all those New England virtues, peculiarly including the one that makes spending money physically painful and the wearing of ancient clothes and fixing of equipment a spiritual lift. Harry owns one sweater. What a curse! Does he have any notion how long he is going to be dead? Wake up, Harry! Get some decent stuff!

Good gear is not a "toy," as a cruel and sneering wife might say; it is lifesaving machinery. And yours will be the life it saves. *Yeats* should rest in a glass case in the middle of

the living room with a brass plaque on the side: IN CASE OF
AGING OR DESPAIR . . . BREAK GLASS! . . . CLIMB ABOARD! For
some amusing dope on good, new gear, go to our Web site,
www.youngernextyear.com.

The High-Endurance Vacation

The more familiar kedge is the killer trip. Again, I particularly recommend biking and skiing. Or hiking or kayaking. But set it up to be tough enough to make it a real
kedge. A while ago I went to a weeklong bike training school
in Barcelona that was a fair model of this kind of thing. It
boasted "serious training and serious fun," which is just what
a kedging trip ought to be. There was some serious training
by some real pros, including the reigning U.S. women's biking champion. She knew a thing or two and she looked like
a sturdier Gwyneth Paltrow, which was okay. There were
beautiful eighty- to hundred-mile rides in the steep hills
above Barcelona and along one of the prettiest coastlines in
the world. There were two hundred Swiss cyclists in the
camp, plus some Swiss instructors, who were not uniformly
amusing. But I learned some neat stuff (take full breaths even
when you feel like panting; it makes the oxygen exchange
more efficient and visibly lowers your heart rate), and I had
long hours of heavy biking all week long. There is nothing
like that to spike and inspire your daily workouts for the next
few months. And don't think you have to go to Spain; loads
of similar opportunities are available locally.

I did another trip, Ride the Rockies, with an old pal and
my godson this June. That's a six-day bike trip, sponsored
by a Denver paper, up and down the Continental Divide in
Colorado. I've done a bunch of these, and they are my all-time

favorite kedge. They are cheap as dirt, and super exercise. Some two thousand people bike as much as 100 miles a day, over 12,000-foot passes (Loveland! Rabbit Ears Pass! Estes Park! names to conjure with), and camp at night in schools and gyms. A huge truck carries your luggage and sleeping bag from site to site. Wonderful biking. Wonderful camaraderie. This is *major*. The prospect of trips like this one and the one to Spain sit in your head for months in advance and for years afterwards. They focus your training and keep you going. And they're great fun.

A Bad Trip

Well, fairly great fun. Be flexible in your expectations, because, as I discovered last winter, it is possible to err. To get hurt. Humiliated. Ashamed. Here's the heartbreaking story. Last summer, a pal named Cheeb, whom I've known since first grade, called to say he had an idea for the book: I should join him for his annual Masters ski racing clinic in Stowe, Vermont, in December. I could report on old boys at play, sharpen my skiing skills and have something to get in shape for. Fine. These things all sound fine, six months in advance.

I hadn't been to Stowe for thirty years, since I discovered western skiing, and kind of wanted to go back now that I thought I was hot. Not Cheeb-level hot, but better than I'd been in 1970; I wanted to show off to the ghost of my old self. Besides, I had relatives up there. Sort of. A Quaker branch of Mother's family had farmed in Stowe for a hundred years before anyone thought about skiing. I had met the last of them, the three "Bigelow girls," when Mother drove us up there in September of 1941 in her green La Salle.

I loved that trip. Mother talking about Eliachim Bigelow (Uncle Like) mowing the fields with a yoke of oxen when she was a kid in the 1890s. Me getting a lesson in milking cows (I can still feel that cow's udder in my nervous hand, even though I haven't touched one in sixty-five years). And the Bigelow Girls, quilting, arguing and "thee-ing and thou-ing" each other in Quaker-speak on the plain covered porch. "Suzie! Where is thy echustechon?" That's an *ear trumpet*. (Think of it: I saw a woman use an *ear trumpet*.) The girls would all be in the little cemetery now, behind the big white church in the middle of town, but that was okay. The farm would still be there. I could go see that. And I would stop by the cemetery and pay my respects.

I had only seen the farm a couple of times, but it was oddly important to me. Mother, who had gone there often as a little girl, talked about it all the time. And the Bigelow Girls, who helped raise her, had lived there all their lives. That lovely old farmhouse, looking out over the Green Mountains, and a half-dozen farms like it in Danvers and Tiverton and Nantucket, which I had only heard about . . . they purred away in memory, just below the surface. Made me feel a little less scared in this hectic world as we go rack-eting along toward . . . some damn thing.

The cemetery was covered with snow. I never found the farm. And the ski part wasn't so great, either: it was scary and shaming. The hitch was Cheeb and his little pals. They were very serious ski racers. I do not mean "Last one to the bottom is a rotten egg!" I mean Masters racing. With gates. And strange costumes. And danger.

At some level, I had known this, and as the time came closer I tried to back out. I was not in good enough shape, I said. I'd been sick. I'd been traveling. The dog had eaten my homework. I told Hilary, and she said, good, she'd been afraid I'd get hurt.

"Oh," I said stupidly, "that's not it. It's the embarrassment. I'll look like an idiot."

Hilary paused for exactly one second. "You mean you're quitting because you're going to be embarrassed?"

I said petulantly that I wasn't "quitting"; I just wasn't starting. Because I had been sick. And maybe a little fat. Not in truly great shape.

"But this whole book," she said, "is you and Harry dragging these poor men out of their La-Z-Boys to gyms, where they're going to be embarrassed for months. And you're staying home because you might be embarrassed for five days? That's appalling!"

Yap, yap, yap. Then she called Harry and he piled right on. The toad. "If that's really it," he said when I took the phone, "I think that's a little raw. Besides, if you were humiliated some, it might be terrific for the book. Hilary's right that we may be a bit haughty here and there. This might be good for you."

"For *me*! What about you! There's no creature on earth haughtier than a nice warm doctor prescribing outdoor exercise for some fat, terrified old gentleman who wants nothing more than to sit and watch TV. If we need to be chastened, why don't *you* go to the stinking race camp?"

"Can't," Harry said serenely. "Too young. And I have a day job, as you know. Besides, it's not that you're that much haughtier than me . . ." He paused as he thought about that for a moment. "It's for the book in general. For both of us, really. And the reader. Very humanizing."

"I don't *need* humanizing, for God's sake. It's the one trait I have in abundance. *You* go." And so on. But of course he couldn't. Or wouldn't. He and Hilary were a wall against me. I sent in the check. And desperately tried to get in shape in three short weeks.

Let me tell you just a little bit about the training effort. It's pretty dull, but it does tell you a couple of things you should maybe know about cross-training, warming up and virtuous stuff like that. To begin with, I started exactly the wrong way by trying to do too much. I wasn't in bad shape, obviously, but not quite ready for a Masters ski racing camp. Masters-level skiers are a different breed. So I leapt into a high-intensity conditioning class with lots and lots of quad-crushing crouches, leaps and push-ups. When I joined the other boys and girls in class (none over thirty-five in this little cadre of killers), they'd been doing it for months. I thought, hell, I've been using my quads, hard, for years now. No problem.

Problem. It's the same muscles, but apparently you come at them a different way and they aren't ready. Biking and spinning are great, but they strengthen your legs in a narrow band. I was now outside that band. Way outside. It was kind of fun for a while. We'd leap over a nine-inch step and down into a deep crouch, our palms touching the floor, way off to one side. Then, quick, leap across the step into the same crouch, on the other side. Then do it again. About twenty times. Well . . . okay. I did that. But that took about two minutes and this was an hour-long class. It got much, much worse. One little number I remember: jump up in the air ten times, then immediately throw yourself on the floor and do a matching set of ten push-ups. It just happens that, today, I can do ten pathetic push-ups . . . a miraculous improvement over five years ago when I couldn't do any. But that turned out to be an introductory bit of fun. Now do nine jumps. Now nine push-ups. And so on. And when you get to one, soaked in sweat and blood, do you quit? Not a bit of it. Go back to ten. Repeat entire progression five times.

I could not "repeat entire progression" once. So I stood there and watched, like a bull that has been cut a little too deep by the picadors. I had to quit long before they were done. It wasn't the aerobics, interestingly. It was the muscles. They were screaming.

I was crippled for days. Crippled so badly that it hurt to walk. Hell, it hurt to sleep. Okay, three lessons for all of us: One, if you're an old boy, don't go into a new sport or training activity at full bore. Let your muscles get used to it, even if you're in decent shape. Two, do some cross-training as a regular part of your routine, so you'll have some range and flexibility. Three, when you throw that kedging anchor into the ocean, let go before it hits the water or it will pull you to the bottom.

Going to Stowe: Real Men (and Women) at Play

A Masters ski racing clinic is a coming together of fifty or sixty crazy people, in this case New Englanders aged forty-five to eighty-eight (sic), who are fond of ski racing. Terminally fond of ski racing. You are familiar, are you not, with the famous distinction between chalk and cheese? Well, the recreational skier (me) is as much like the racing skier (these birds) as chalk is like cheese. I had no more business in a Masters ski racing clinic than a golden retriever. For one thing, I am a rational man. Ski racers are crazy as loons.

Consider the scene on the third and worst day of camp. It is 7:45 in the warm-up hut near the gondola. This is *eastern* skiing. The warm-up hut is a huge, Spartan shed of the type used in Aspen to shelter heavy machinery or large pets. There is a tiny commissary where nasty food is sold at low prices that would be astonishing if the food were edible, which it is not. That does not matter because the good folk who ski here are New Englanders, and they bring their own lunch in brown paper bags. Which they fold up and reuse, day after day. Their food is nasty, too, but at least they don't have to pay for it. They don't care about food anyway; they care about skiing. They care too much. It snowed a lot yesterday, but today rain is expected. Most of these folks have brought huge garbage bags in which to ski when rain really starts to come down. I do not have a garbage bag. I will not need it.

At one end of the shed, my new friends are putting on their things so they can be on the slopes by 8:00, when it may be daylight. I have been skiing most of my life and am familiar with many of its little rituals, but there are some new things going on here. Not just the garbage bags. Worse. Much worse.

A group of nice-looking old ladies, in their mid to late sixties, are matter-of-factly strapping hard plastic protectors to their shins. Others are calmly strapping similar gear to their forearms. I am a bit of an equipment freak, and there is very little ski equipment of which I do not own several versions. I have never seen these things before. I have never *heard* of them. I learn that it is called "armor" and is favored by slalom racers all over the world. It is so basic, indeed, that one little old lady, who has left hers at home, is quietly cutting pieces off a big cardboard box with her own Leatherman knife and shaping them into homemade armor. She fits the cardboard to her shins and straps it on with duct tape. Which she happens to have with her. I feel ill.

An eighty-six-year-old man sits in a corner fooling with his helmet with *his* Leatherman. He is making sure that the face guard is securely screwed on. I have never seen a face guard on a ski helmet. Every person in the room but me has one. What is this madness? I ask Cheeb plaintively. Why are we in this grim room, in the dark, with these elderly lunatics? And what are they doing?

We are here, Cheeb explains cheerfully, and they are dressing up, because this is "slalom day." You, Chris, may be going a bit slower and will not have a problem, but these sexa-, septua- and octogenarians will be flying down the ice ruts and will want to protect themselves as they deliberately crash over the slalom poles that indicate where they are to turn. It develops that these poles, which obstruct the reasonable route down the hill, are on springs or gimbals, and can be knocked down by the sturdier skier. Only the ski boots of these people will be on the "right" side of the poles. The rest of their screaming, wrinkled bodies will be canted dangerously over the poles, which must of course be gotten out of the way. So they'll smack them smartly with their arms, lower legs, jaws or what have you. It is what they like. They look forward to the day.

I do not. I wish to go to my home, and I suggest to Cheeb that this might make sense. No, says Cheeb, you'll do fine. I've seen you ski for two days, and you'll be fine.

Well, that was a little lie. I did do it. I went tearing down the dear old mountain at what seemed to me breakneck speed, screaming into and out of the icy ruts, smacking into the terrible poles (occasionally) and often shooting out of the course completely and heading for the woods. I was scared, clumsy and embarrassed the whole day. Just as I'd known I would be. You cannot conceive how dangerous and unpleasant it is to ski a tight series of deep, ice-walled ruts, even at modest speeds, under the highly critical eye of people who have been doing it, on purpose, for fifty or sixty years. Never, never again.

But there were some wonderful things.

These people—many in their sixties but a good many in their seventies and eighties—were beautiful skiers. There was one elegant, sixty-five-year-old woman who had been first alternate for the 1960 Olympics and, believe me, she looked it. And the three men in their eighties . . . I could not believe how lithe they were. Not creaking along, not taking a last run for old times' sake. But skiing hard, with obvious pleasure. There was one woman—perhaps in her late fifties—who was one of the most beautiful skiers I've ever seen. A tall, handsome Scandinavian, she went sloping through those gates with incredible grace. Cheeb said she looks exactly the same at fifty miles an hour, which she hits routinely. I have never skied fifty miles an hour and don't intend to. But I might go back to see her do it.

Another reason I might *conceivably* go back, perhaps for a day or two, is that I have never learned so much, so fast. Terrific racing instructors helped a lot, but mostly it was my fellow skiers. They *all* felt free to give pointers to someone as clueless as me. The way grown-ups used to feel free to lecture everybody's children when I was little. One of the old ladies rounded on me sharply and said, "For God's sake, get your feet apart!" "I have got my feet apart!" I whined. "Oh, puh-leeze," she snorted. "Like this!" And off she sailed. Turns out that she was the near-Olympian. So I spread my legs a little.

One night, in a modest "chalet" with deep roots in the 1950s, there was a cocktail party—a Vermont cocktail party with five different kinds of potato chips and a dip made from dehydrated onion soup. It was fun. The group, a club of Masters racers who have been together for twenty years, knew and liked each other well. There was lots of ski talk, lots of race talk and lots and lots of old-pal gossip. Good scene. We talk later in the book about the need to make new connections (and keep old ones) as you get older. These men and women had that project well in hand. That's a basic life tip, by the way: Make a sports or athletic group—like your bike or swim pals—into a "connect and commit" support group. Like a book group, only stronger. And weirder.

Talk about life-affirming! There was one handsome old gent whose brand-new wife had just joined the group. They were both serious skiers and absolutely blooming about their new life together. John was eighty-eight and his new wife was eighty-five; they looked and sounded to be in their early sixties. Cheeb told John that I had lived in Aspen for a while, and he was immediately curious. Turns out he had an interesting stake in Aspen. He was there the day it was invented. He had been in the fabled 10th Mountain Division at Camp Hale during World War II, one of the ski troopers who had fought ferociously in the Italian mountains and then become the founding fathers of skiing in America. This man had led a group on overnight maneuvers from Camp Hale to what was then the dying mining town of Aspen. One of his troopers was the young (later legendary) Friedl Pfeiffer, who said, "This would be a great ski town. I'm coming back after the war." He did, and the rest is skiing history. That probably doesn't do much for you, but it gave me goose bumps.

On the fourth day, I got a massive break. It snowed. A lot. Two feet, easy. A near record in this ice-hell. And it was powder, too, not the usual eastern muck. You cannot run races in that much snow, so school was out and we had a day of free play. Now, those old giants can ski anything, most assuredly including powder, but it was a bit of an equalizer. We skied until it was almost dark, rejoicing in the powder like madmen. Including two of the eighty-year-olds, right down to the last run. I cannot tell you what a kick it was to go flying down those hills in deep powder, side by side with those people.

Okay, there are a couple of morals to be drawn. Doing stuff that scares the hell out of you—or embarrasses you or makes you feel like a dope—does have a place. In most cases it can't kill you, and the learning curve can be exhilaratingly steep. It opens your head up at an age when you're tempted to shut it down. Besides, scary is memorable. One of the curses of getting older is that time speeds up and the days seem much the same. Well, you want to slow time down? Remember some things? Go to race camp if you're not a racer. Go on a long bike ride if you're not a biker. I will remember that week in Stowe, clearly, until the day I die.

Last point: role models. I do not for a minute suggest that what real athletes like Cheeb and his pals do "informs" the lives of simple folk like you and me. But it is still true that three octogenarians were out there skiing. They did not all look great all the time, but they looked pretty damn good. And they were *out there*. That's the point. My goal? I don't want to be a Masters skier, but I sure want to be out there. When I'm eighty-five. Or ninety. And I want you to be out there, too.

Come to think of it, "going for it" is what kedging is all about. There are as many kedging trips and kedging devices as there are good ideas, and that's infinite. But the one unifying theme is this: Make it serious, make it fun. And go for it.

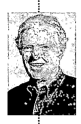

CHAPTER TEN

A World of Pain: Strength Training

How many times has someone slid up to you and said, "Hey, I've got a neat idea! Let's go down to the gym and lift incredibly heavy weights until it hurts like crazy and we have to stop!" Once a week? Once a year? Let me guess. Never? And why is that? Because lifting weights is stupid, embarrassing and painful, that's why.

I remember the first time I decided to venture into a weight room. It was when I lived in Aspen, where they tend to hide weight rooms in "spas," which look deceptively normal at street level. Lots of expensive shrubbery, lots of glass. A pretty girl just inside the door to take your dough and sign you up for a year. It happens very fast. The pretty girl takes your credit card and says, "I'm Chanterelle, by the way. Let me show you the pool." Which she does. It's nice. Then the cheerful room full of aerobic dancers. The step machines and the stationary bicycles. Nice. It all looks nice.

Then you get down to business: "So, look, do you, uh
. . . have a weight room?"

A cloud passes over Chanterelle's face. "Sure, sure. Let's
go take a look." A hurried glance back at the counter and the
mouthed words "Run his card!" Then down the rubber steps
into an underground space that looks like a cross between the
engine room of an old destroyer and a dominatrix's mud-
room. Lots of tile and mirrors. Drains in the floor, so it can
be hosed down when they're done with you. Huge steel
machines with black pads all over. Lifting machines, twisting
machines . . . machines to pull the teeth out of a Caterpillar
tractor. And lots of sleek wires connecting this and that.
Wires that seem to be used to tie up pretty girls, who struggle to get free, with a tremendous amount of sweat and not
much luck. Young men, too. Men with weird veins running
all over their arms and necks. Like fat worms under the skin.
Veins like macaroni on acid and biceps that look as if they've
been blown out. This is a scary place.

"Listen, you probably have a lot to do. I'll just—"

"No, no," Chanterelle says quickly. "You've already
paid. You're dressed. Let me just get Lance. Oh, Lance . . ."

Up hulks this guy with a deep tan and more teeth than
you've ever seen in one mouth before. Sort of nice-looking,
but something's terribly wrong. Like his body doesn't quite
make sense. And the planes of his face . . . they're way too
sharp. This guy is . . .

Lance (or Biff or Hawk) says, "Hi, let me show you
around," and begins this rap about the machines and his special training techniques. But you're not listening . . . you're
just staring, nervously. At his body. Because it's becoming
clear to you that he is almost certainly an android. And the
manufacturer has scrimped on the little life-giving details
that are so important. Maybe a foreign manufacturer, too,

because he's dressed funny. His little red shorts look much too small on his huge thighs. And he's wearing a sleeveless T-shirt with enormous armholes through which it is impossible not to see his pecs, or whatever they're called. And his armpits. His armpits are the deepest and furriest you have ever seen. You could raise wolverines in there. You want to take a step back so he won't drip testosterone all over your sneakers. You want to get the hell out of there . . .

Why, you ask yourself, why is this man telling me all this in a book promoting exercise? I am telling you this because I want to persuade you to find a strength trainer—maybe not as bad as Lance, but bad—and learn to do weights. And then do them two days a week for the rest of your life. And I want you to know that Harry and I realize this is not an intuitively appealing idea. Regular strength training for life sounds stupid, nasty and scary. And we wouldn't even mention it if it were not one of the best pieces of advice in the whole damn book. Strength training will make you feel good and stay healthy for the rest of your life—once you get over the shame and terror and revulsion. In fact, it's so important that Harry has memorialized it in his Third Rule, which goes like this: *Do serious strength training, with weights, two days a week for the rest of your life.*

The Payoff

Do you remember how we talked about the tide that sets against you by the time you're fifty? The tide that threatens to wash you up on the beach where the gulls and the crabs are waiting to do unpleasant things? Lifting weights is one of the critical things you do to stay off the beach. Because of your bones and your muscles and, most importantly, your joints.

Take bone first. In the normal course (and please remember that the "normal course" is no longer your friend), you lose 0.3 to 0.5 percent of your bone mass every year after age forty. That's right, the tide is sucking the bone out of your bones at the rate of perhaps one percent every couple of years. Which is one of the things that turns us into little old guys, all bent over and stupid-looking. Fall down, break your hip. Go to bed. Never get up.

And muscle mass. That goes, too. Out with the tide. Turning the sweet muscles of your youth into the dusty drapery of old age. Makes you too weak to do stuff. Like run across the street if you have to. Or get out of the tub. Or ski. Or make love . . . move your pelvis back and forth in that pleasing way. No matter what, you're going to lose muscle cells as you age; that's one of the things you cannot change.

Your joints—the meshing bones and the tendons and sinews and goopy pads that make them work—are even more important at your age because they go to hell first if you don't do something. The little grippers that attach tendon to bone get brittle and weak as you age. They atrophy. They let go without notice. And the goopy pads between the bones dry out and you make little crunching sounds when you move. And you hurt. The combination of all this stuff is aging joints, and it has more to do with your aging than almost anything else. When your joints go, you hurt all the time. You walk funny. You fall down. You get old.

Sounds bad, right? Well, here's the weird thing. Lifting big, heavy weights stops most of that. Lifting heavy weights every couple of days basically stops the bone loss . . . stops (or offsets) the muscle loss . . . stops the weakening of tendons, restores the goopy pads and gets rid of the pain. Aerobic exercise does more to stop actual death, but strength training can make your life worthwhile. It keeps your muscle mass from going to muck, your skeleton from turning to dust, your joints from hurting with every lousy step. This is key. We would not put you through the horror of weight training if it were not key. Here's another odd thing. After you've been doing it for a while, you kind of get into it. We'll come back to that.

Hire a Trainer or
Read a Book or Both

So what do you do? Hire a trainer, at least to get started. Trainers are expensive, Lord knows, but they're worth it. Learning to do weights is a little harder than it looks, and a surprising number of people you see in the gym are doing it wrong. Doing it wrong is both counterproductive and dangerous. Not "kill you" dangerous, but "hurt your joints and drive you away" dangerous. So hire a trainer for the first few workouts. And go back to him or her once in a while to keep yourself honest. Besides, for most of us, the world of weight lifting is such a strange land that it doesn't hurt to have a friendly guide to get you past the weirdness.

If money is an issue—money is *always* an issue—you can get started by reading a decent book on the subject. There are any number of books that offer good guidance and neat little drawings or photos of guys doing stuff. But stay away from the books that promise to do it all for you in five minutes a week or some such nonsense. And avoid the temptation to buy one of those snappy gadgets on TV that promise to do all the work, without any unpleasant input from you. You're a grown-up, right? Then don't be a dope. *The gadgets, or the weights, do not do the work. You do*. If you could mail it in, we'd all look like the guy in the TV ads.

Okay, go to a decent gym and hire the nicest, smartest man or woman you can find. I was mostly kidding about Lance. There are guys like that out there—lots of them, actually. But there are plenty of informed people who are seriously interested in how bodies work and in making yours work better. It's a hot little field these days, and good guys are going into it. I swear by a man in New York who does look a teeny bit like an android but who, in fact, knows this stuff cold and cares passionately about how I'm doing. That's what you want.

Do not make the mistake of hiring some person who just talks to you. Or listens. The gyms are full of people paying big bucks to have guys chat with them and occasionally hand them a weight. You want someone serious who will teach you to do it right and, in time, get you to do it hard. You want someone who can tell you about range of motion and the right pace for a given set of repetitions. Doing reps fast is very tempting, but it's always a bad idea. You need someone to *make* you slow down. And to keep doing reps when you want to quit. A good trainer does that and a lot more.

Some Training Tips

Harry and I are not the ones to tell you what machines or free weights to use and how to do it; we leave that to your trainer and the books. But we do have a couple of points. First: You are forty, or fifty, or sixty . . . you are not twenty or thirty. Second: You are here to be younger *next year*, not next week. You don't want to make a mess of things in the first few days. So, much as it runs against my temperament to say it, take it easy. If you're one of the handful of men your age who's in great shape, take it *sort of* easy. If you're like the rest of us, take it *really* easy. In the next chapter, Harry will tell you that you can build muscle pretty quickly, even at your age, but joints take much, much longer. Strong muscles can pull weak joints apart. So, in the first few months, do less weight than you can handle and more reps—maybe twenty instead of the usual ten or twelve. Give your joints time to get in the game.

Light weights and high reps in the beginning make sense for another reason: muscle memory. You may not think it, but using weights is a little like learning a new sport—not as complex as skiing or tennis, but a new sport just the same. And your muscles have to learn how. That's less true with the machines, which is why free weights are better for you. They involve balancing and subtle corrections from side to side, all of which use and strengthen a whole bunch of other muscles and, more important, zillions of neuroconnectors, which are at the heart of your ability to function in the real world. It's not just the strength that matters, it's the *wiring*, too. The amazing message system that tells you where you are in the world and lets you function. By all means, use machines to get started and mix machines into your strength training indefinitely, but get into free weights, too.

Don't show off. Guys are irresistibly tempted to pick up the heaviest weights they can find and totter around under them, proud as six-year-olds. Don't. It's silly and dangerous. And whatever your DNA tells you about competing with the other males in the pack for girls, it doesn't really work that way anymore. Besides, you'll hurt yourself. *Don't swing your weights, either,* in a desperate effort to do more. That's the cardinal sin of weight lifting, and you see it all the time. It does less to make you strong—and more to wreck your joints—than anything else. Ask your trainer. Read your book.

But do not swing weights that are too heavy for you in an effort to look like more of a guy.

Eventually you have to get to heavy weights and low reps. You have to do weights "to failure" some of the time. That means pain. That means lifting weight that you can lift, say, only ten times before you literally cannot do it anymore. Sounds nasty, doesn't it? But bear in mind how this process works. You build muscle by tearing it down. It's all part of the growth and decay business that Harry is teaching us about. You actually tear the muscles a little by lifting heavy weights. When they grow back, they're bigger and stronger. Your bone mass increases at the same time. And you gain tendon strength. And neuroconnector strength, which may be the most important of all.

To make real progress on the strength front, you may have to go to three days a week. (My trainer says two days is for maintenance, three days is for getting stronger.) If you do go to three days, rotate the areas covered. Your muscles need a day, or even two days, to recover from a serious weight session. If you don't rest between sessions, it's all teardown and no buildup. Not good. And don't forget aerobics. No matter what, you have to have at least four days of aerobics each week.

Some weight room guys get aerobics in during their weight-lifting days by going on a fast "circuit." That is, they rush from one set of reps to another—and from machine to machine—with little rest in between in order to get an aerobic as well as a strength workout. I guess that's okay. By the time you get to circuit training with weights, you presumably have a pretty good idea about what you're doing. But be sure you get a serious aerobic workout, one way or another, for forty-five minutes a day, four days a week. It is indispensable.

Default to Quads

If you run out of time (or passion) for doing weights, do whatever you can for your legs, especially your quads. This means squats, or one of those big machines where you sit down and push a weighted sled up a ramp with your legs. Or any of several other machines and exercises aimed primarily at your quads. Do your hamstrings, too, maybe using the machine that makes you pull back with your heels.

A lot of men default to using barbells for their biceps or bench presses for their chests, and forget their legs. Not smart. When your legs give out, you're cooked. That means the cane, the walker and the chair. Nothing is more important than heading that off. And nothing helps more than doing serious weights with your quads and hamstrings.

· Strengthening your quads is also the best thing you can do to prevent bad knees. Strengthening your quads, the shock absorbers of your body, means you're much less likely to fall and get injured. And strengthening your quads, the biggest muscles in your body, means they will burn more calories, even on "idle." And the more testosterone they will generate. So, when in doubt, default to quads.

The Nursing Home Miracle and Other Payoff Stories

It's never too late to start a serious program of strength training. Quite the contrary. The later in life, the more important it is. There was a study done a while ago in a nursing home. They got all the residents, including the ones who were on walkers or bedridden, to do weights. It worked miracles, even though some of these people were in their nineties. Almost all the bedridden got up on walkers. The guys on walkers went to canes, and so on. Moral: Weight training is serious therapy to halt or reverse the ravages of aging. Do it early and you can skip a lot of aging altogether. Do it late and you can reverse a lot of it. I have felt those results myself, big time.

Here's another little payoff story from a couple of months ago. It was 15 degrees, early in the morning in New York, and I was down by the East River, walking Aengus, the selfish dog. Bright sun, wind on the river. And all of a sudden I felt like running. Not for exercise or to show off (no one was around) . . . just for the hell of it. And I did. Cutting this way and that like a hundred-year-old football player. Astonishing the dog, who joined right in. Strange. Nice. I remembered, later, a time a year ago when Aengus was running around on the lawn like that. Like a lunatic. I said to Hilary then, "Gee, I wish I felt like doing that." And here I was, running around like a lunatic, out of sheer exuberance. Because I felt like it.

Strength training does that for you. It makes you look a little better, too. Not great, mind you. You're still an old numero. But if you're in shape, you can take off your clothes at night and look very similar to a human being as you climb into bed. Not like a fat old plop that no one wants to sleep with. It's worth the pain, gents, worth the pain.

Don't worry too much about muscle mass. The object of weight training at this point in your life is not to look like a bodybuilder, but to keep your joints supple, your bones solid and your muscles okay. Besides, there is a surprisingly imperfect correlation between visible muscle mass and strength. You want to be reasonably strong; you do not necessarily want to be big. The ideal physique for the endurance athlete is lithe and lean, and you are an endurance athlete these days.

Speaking of muscle mass, there was a famous movie, about a hundred years ago, called *Pumping Iron,* starring

Arnold Schwarzenegger. The movie led to a bit of a vogue in weight lifting. But the real hype came when the star—long before he was an actor *or* the governor of California—said on *The Late Show,* "A good pump is like coming." What? Suddenly, gyms had lines out the door and weight trainers were stars. I do not know what Arnold's sex life was like, but I hope it was better than my weight-training life. Still, I have to admit—with shy shame—that there is something oddly seductive about a good pump. I actually find myself looking forward to it and enjoying it, ever so slightly, while it's going on. Not to the point of orgasm yet, but, hey . . . who knows?

Until your sex life takes that odd turn, the real reward for lifting is feeling great the rest of the time, when you're just walking around. Especially in your joints. That reward isn't instantaneous—it can take months—but it's a big deal. In my case, when I took this up seriously, I had a lot of sore joints: hips, shoulders, elbows, wrists, Achilles tendon . . . the works. I was starting to totter around like a little old guy, even though I did a fair amount of aerobic activity. It was creepy. I was going to an odd, sidearm tennis serve, which was useless and made me look a hundred. Sometimes just reaching for something on a shelf gave me a little twinge. Aging. I was aging. And you will, too. Unless . . .

When I started weights, *all that went away*! Not my arthritic hands, but the rest of it. I am not exaggerating. I remember how I used to creak and wobble and hurt a little, first trip down the stairs in the morning. *Gone!* My hips do not hurt anymore. Or my feet. Not even my shoulders, which were the worst and took the longest. My serve still stinks, but it's no longer sidearm. Even my Achilles tendon, which I wrecked in 1982 and suffered with for decades, has responded and I've been able to start running again. All because of weights. Harry warns that some of my aches will come back as I get older, but not for quite a while and not as bad. I'll take that.

Part of what I was curing was mild arthritis, which is nothing more than inflammation, often brought on by idleness. So when some of my pals say they can't do weights because they have arthritis and it hurts, I tell them they probably hurt and have arthritis because they don't do weights. Consider the fact that, for most forms of arthritis, the prescription is a six-week course of physical therapy. Guess what? Physical therapy is, in large part, nothing more than supervised weight training. You should not just be doing it for six weeks, which is when your insurance usually runs out. You should be doing it for life, two times a week. It will do more than anything else to prevent most forms of arthritis if you don't already have it. And to make it better if you do.

Here's another huge change: I quit falling down. One of the truly alarming things that happened in my early sixties was that I began falling for no reason at all. Two or three times, I was crossing the street or just walking on a city sidewalk and stumbled over a little uneven place or a rise in the pavement. I'd catch the bottom of my sneaker and go flying, as if I'd forgotten how to walk. And I wasn't even *old*. I was in decent shape and pretty damn active, but I was falling down. Man, talk about hearing the waterfall. I thought I was going over.

Once I was carrying a lot of stuff and had Aengus on a lead, running across Park Avenue as the light was about to change. I caught the bottom of my foot on the pavement, and down I went. The light changed, and I was in the middle of the cars. Aengus was loose and terrified. I was dazed and surrounded by broken packages. Horns were honking, and a woman in the median actually screamed because she thought I was going to be killed. I thought so, too.

Something similar happened on a mountain hike out west, ten years ago. The steep part, the challenging part, was over, and that had gone fine. Now we were on the flat, half a mile from the parking lot, and for no reason I tripped and tumbled off the trail. Landed on top of my own leg and broke it. Was put into a cast and couldn't exercise all summer. I thought, so this is aging. Great!

The happy fact is that it did not have to be that way, and it isn't anymore. The reason I was falling, Harry tells me, is that the neurotransmitters that coordinate balance deteriorate with age. Which is to say, your balance goes and you walk into stuff as if you were an idiot. Harry says that, for all of us, simple walking is really a series of near falls followed by a million tiny adjustments and recovery. When you age, the wiring that manages that stunt falls apart, and so do you. You no longer catch yourself. And here, of course, is the pleasing news. Lifting weights fixes up the wiring and cures the problem. Not a hundred percent, Harry says, but damn near. In my experience, anyway. I have not fallen in years. Don't even stumble much, or come close. Presumably because I do the stinking weights. I tell you, I swear by 'em. Try it.

Luckily, you do not have to take all this on faith or in reliance on one old boy's experience. Harry is going to explain the science, and All Will Be Made Clear, in the next chapter. To me, it's holy writ. I didn't much like all that falling down.

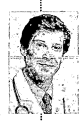

CHAPTER ELEVEN

The Biology of Strength Training

A erobic exercise is primarily about your muscles' ability to endure. Strength training is primarily about your muscles' ability to deliver power, which, surprisingly, has as much to do with a special form of neural coordination as actual strength. That's a critical point. Strength training causes muscle growth, and that's important, but it's the hidden increase in coordination that changes your physical life. This is not eye-hand coordination; it's the coordination of fine muscle detail through the elaborate networks of nerves that link your brain and body.

Generally, we aren't aware of nerve decay as we get older, but it's the main reason our joints wear out, our muscles get sloppy and our ability to be physically alert and powerful begins to fade. And it is reversible with strength training.

It's easier to illustrate how this works by example, so let's look at what happens when you take a single step up a single stair. That might sound too simple, but in my first year of medical school I sat through a two-hour lecture on the neural coordination required to swallow a single bite of food.

A Single Step

Think about how much play your knee tolerates in simple walking: the moderate amount of bending and jarring you subject it to during each step. Now imagine standing at the foot of a flight of stairs. Climb the stairs in slow motion, two at a time. Notice that your thigh and calf contract, hard, at the very beginning of each step, and the first thing this does is pull the knee joint instantly into a very tight alignment *before you actually move.*

You might think this is just the result of tightening all the muscles simultaneously, and you are partly right, but it is also critically important that each muscle tighten to just the right degree to put your joints in perfect alignment to do the mechanical work you're asking of it. A mechanic tightens the fan belt on your car to a specific tolerance and then bolts it in place. Your body is far more sophisticated, and adjusts the fan belt for maximum efficiency and safety with each step. Each joint is automatically pre-tensioned to just the right position for each step.

Now hold this book out in front of you with both hands and stand up slowly. Focus on the precise delivery of power from your muscles throughout the motion. It involves all the major muscle groups in your lower back, buttocks, thighs, calves and feet, as well as a host of minor, stabilizing muscle groups in your spine, torso, shoulders, abdomen and pelvis. Seriously, stand up from your chair in slow motion, noting the muscles involved from your head to your toes.

You go through these coordinated cycles tens of thousands of times in the average day. Each step, each coordinated movement, involves thousands of nerve fibers, which together form a neural network. You have millions of potential neural networks in your body, and you shift between them with each step. Your body grows and your brain learns the tiniest amount from each one. They have to, because C-6 is in the background, helping them to forget all this, just a little bit, every day.

The trouble comes when your muscles, brain connections and the controlling spinal reflex arcs get sloppy and weak from years of a relatively sedentary existence. The casual motion of daily life is not enough to turn on the C-10 of growth. Pushing your chair back from the desk is an insultingly trivial task for your physical brain, and over the decades large parts of it have deliberately gone to sleep in protest. Remember the threshold for C-10? It takes a critical amount of effort to cross that threshold and secrete enough C-6 to trigger the production of C-10. Below that threshold, all you have is the C-6 of chronic decay. You need to do strength training to cross that threshold for power and coordination, to get C-10 into your neural networks, into the meat of your muscles, into your joints and into your tendons.

Aerobic exercise takes you across the threshold for endurance, circulation and longevity, but you need strength training for power and neural coordination. A single step on level ground doesn't turn on C-10. Nor does climbing a few stairs. But climbing stairs until you feel your legs burn will turn on C-10. Lifting weights until you can't lift them anymore . . . that *really* turns on C-10.

The Brain-Body Connection

Strength training creates an intimate connection between your body and your brain. It's easiest to look at this from the top down, starting with your brain and nervous system. Your physical brain—the remarkably complex, physical brain—integrates the millions of messages coming up from your body and coordinates them with all the impulses it's sending down to move your muscles against resistance. The neural impulses to create coordination and power blaze a trail through your neural circuits. Each time you use them, you directly strengthen the balance, power and muscular coordination centers of the physical brain. And the trail gets broader, smoother and faster.

Athletes have come to realize the benefits of strength training over the last thirty years. But the interesting thing is that the greatest advances have come not in the strength sports, like the shot put and weight lifting, but in the coordination sports—the ones that require grace, skill and coordination, like figure skating and skiing. Those improvements are due largely to increased coordination and muscular integration, as well as the increased muscle power available for jumping and landing, developed through strength training. The same can be true for you. You still have the circuitry to do a triple jump on skates or, more realistically, to run across the court and hit a powerful backhand, but it's a shadow of what it could be. Indeed, the last time most of us used these neural connections to their full extent was during fourth-grade recess.

Consistent strength training can change all that by bringing your neural connections out of hibernation. For example, even though it *feels* as if you're contracting 100 percent of each muscle involved in level walking, only 10 percent of the cells in those muscles are actually in use. These cells are distributed evenly throughout each muscle, so every part of it moves, but 90 percent of the cells are resting . . . going along for the ride. With harder exercise, you recruit an increasing number of cells. Walking up a real hill or a long flight of stairs, you might use 30 percent of the muscle cells during a given step. Lifting the heaviest weight you can handle, you might even use half the muscle cells at once, but that's about it.

The ability to choose which muscle cells get activated— and the degree of contraction—gives us an amazing physical potential. Running across a tennis court to hit a forehand requires subtle shades of coordination for the direction, arc, spin and force of the shot—which means that each of the muscles in your legs and arm has to play its own part in a simultaneous symphony. Hundreds of thousands of nerve cells, controlling hundreds of millions of muscle cells. A massive harmony that lasts a split second, just to hit a ball across a net. That's the neural information superhighway we talked about earlier—the billions of nerve signals flying around your body every minute of the day.

Slow-Twitch, Fast-Twitch

The nerves that control your muscles contain thousands of individual cells, each of which splits further into hundreds and hundreds of tiny branches. And each branch goes to one—and only one—muscle cell. There are over a million muscle cells in the large muscles of your thighs, and perhaps ten thousand nerve cells, bundled into a couple of main nerves, controlling them all.

This gets detailed, but stick with it. You have two types of muscle cells, built for strength or for endurance, and they are different. This is a critical point, so I'm going to repeat it.

Your muscles have strength cells and endurance cells, and they are different.

Muscle endurance cells are known as slow-twitch. They have more mitochondria, more endurance and less power. Muscle strength cells are known as fast-twitch: fewer mitochondria, less endurance and much more power. Each individual nerve cell sends all of its tentacles to *either* strength *or* endurance cells, but never both. This means that each individual nerve cell ends up signaling for either strength or endurance. Remember that, in your thigh, for instance, each of these nerve cells has thousands of tiny branches, going to thousands of muscle cells, all either strength or endurance. Your quadriceps muscle, the big one in the front of your thigh, has over a million muscle cells. The big nerve that controls it has around ten thousand nerve cells. Each one of those nerve cells controls a few thousand muscle cells, called a motor unit, in a specific pattern.

Now we can look at how you actually move. Your brain can activate any combination of those motor units to perform specific movements. The choices your physical brain makes, instantly, between the thousands of motor units in each muscle are what give you the ability to dance, spin, jump or just wiggle your toes. You activate only a fraction of the nerve cells with each step, but it's a very carefully chosen fraction for each individual muscle. It's a little daunting to think of the complexity of all this, of the millions of split-second decisions your physical brain makes just to keep you on your feet, let alone dancing. Luckily, you don't have to think about it; you can take it for granted. It is vitally important that you understand that it's there, but you can go years without worrying about it if you take care of it.

Chris talks about skiing as a strength sport, which is true enough, but the equally important point is that it's a *coordi-*

nated strength sport. Strength training makes both the power and the coordination possible and delivers them in the integrated package that lets Chris ski well at seventy, and will let you live well at any age.

With this as background, let's look at strength training vs. endurance exercise. When you walk, your body predominantly recruits endurance units and rotates through them so each one gets a rest period between steps, which means that each unit gets only a fraction of the exercise you think you're giving it. Certainly not enough stress to generate the powerful regeneration of C-10.

As you start to run, your body uses more endurance units with each step. Each unit may be used every third step now, and that's enough stress to trigger high levels of C-6 and then C-10. If you're running up a hill, hard enough to go beyond the capacity of your endurance units, your body adds in strength units. The longer you run, the less rest time the endurance units get. The more strength you demand, the less rest the strength units get. At some point, you will push them beyond their recovery cycles. They will fatigue, and the fatigue will damage them. Taking them to fatigue is what turns on the surge of C-6—the good stress of exercise that turns on C-10.

By the way, this is why you have to sweat when you do aerobic exercise; at low levels of demand, your endurance cells alternate too much to get fatigued. This is also why you have to push to the point of muscle fatigue with weights—to that burning feeling in your muscles that most of us hate and would skip if it were up to us.

When you hire that personal trainer, he or she will eventually make sure you lift enough weight to cycle all the way through the reserve capacity of your strength cells. To use them ten or twelve times in a row, and then do it again. Done right, you will drain them of all their energy

Peak Fitness: Who Needs It?

You do not build new muscle cells with strength training; in fact, you continue to slowly lose them as you age, regardless. What you do instead is build new muscle mass inside each remaining cell: the protein, the substance—in short, the red meat. And the potential growth in those remaining cells is extraordinary: certainly enough to keep you strong and fit for the rest of your long life.

Put another way, you can lose half your muscle cells over the course of your life, lose half your peak fitness, and still end up stronger at eighty than you were at twenty. Besides, when were you ever at your peak fitness? No one but Olympic athletes and Navy SEALS ever get there. The current world bench-press record for sixty-year-old men is 440 pounds. The world record for young guys is 700 pounds. Both numbers scare me, but they illustrate a key point. Peak performance declines with age. The guy who can bench 700 pounds at age twenty will be down to 440 pounds by age sixty. That's a 40 percent decline in maximum strength.

Sound pretty grim? Well, it's not. After all, how strong do you need to be? The sixty-year-old can bench-press your refrigerator with you sitting on top of it. He has lost 40 percent of his muscle cells, but look what he's done with the ones he has left! For men over eighty-five, by the way, the world bench-press record is 175 pounds. Which is still more than most of us can do.

and *then* force them to contract a few more times. That's the critical part; that's how you intentionally damage your muscle cells. Not your muscles, just the muscle cells. And you damage them quite a lot. On purpose. Electron microscope pictures of muscle from bodybuilders show extensive damage at the cellular level after a workout. That's fine and what your body needs. Lots of C-6, lots of inflammation, and then lots of repair and growth. Your muscles will quiver and burn, which is not fun, but inside you will be forcing your brain to activate *all* your strength units. Do this for three sets, and you will have forced your body to *damage* all those strength units, which then forces it to *repair* all those strength units. Growth, strength—youth.

This is why you shouldn't do strength training six days a week. If you've done it right, you've done some real damage. Unlike endurance units, which recover from aerobic exercise overnight, your strength units need to enter a forty-eight-hour repair cycle. Two days a week of strength training is enough. Three days is the maximum.

Doing It Right

By the way, you want to be very, very careful not to confuse damaging your muscle cells by *exhausting* them with damaging your muscles or joints by *overloading* them. It's tempting to use heavy weights so you can exhaust the muscle cells with fewer repetitions, because, frankly, the repetitions hurt. They feel lousy, and eight is a lot easier to tolerate than twelve or fifteen. But you are not young. You will be *younger* next year, but you will not be *young* next year. Your trainer will almost certainly be younger than you are and may not understand this in his or her bones, so you are in charge of not getting hurt. Also, as you get into better shape and get stronger, your brain will secrete more adrenaline when you exercise. You will start to enjoy the weights and look forward to going to the gym. The downside is that the adrenaline of strength training will activate your primitive impulse to show off to the other males, to push yourself to your peak performance, where injuries happen. Don't go there.

The Balancing Act

Now it's time to think about your brain and a concept called proprioception—the deceptively simple notion that you have to know where the different parts of your body are at all times. It's how we stand up and how we move. We stand on two feet like a ladder standing straight up into the sky, not leaning against anything. That's an amazing feat on our part. Try balancing a ladder straight up. You have to make constant adjustments to keep it from falling over. Our bodies are just the same. And that's the simple stuff. Try running around the yard holding a ladder straight up. Try to spin around and throw to first base holding the ladder straight up. Try to do any of the amazing things *we* do all the time standing on two feet. And then try it standing on one foot!

Your body is aware of exactly where each limb is in space every second, because each muscle, tendon, ligament and joint sends thousands of nerve fibers back to the brain through the spinal cord. Those fibers signal every nuanced gradation of contraction, strength, muscular tone, orientation, position and movement at every moment of the day. Close your eyes and concentrate on your index finger. You know exactly where it is to within a couple of millimeters, automatically; same thing with your big toe or left elbow. Keep your eyes closed and do a quick survey of where each part of your body is right now. Your brain keeps careful track of the location of every muscle and joint in your body every second, all day, every day, waiting for you to need the information. And it sends millions of signals throughout the day just to keep you upright and aware of where you're standing.

Strength training works on these signals. Pushing a muscle hard sends a blaring signal back up to the brain. Remember adjusting the fan belt, the instant tightening of your joints on the staircase? This is important stuff for your body. If your brain slacks off for an instant, and you don't make the split-second adjustments, you might get hurt. You will pull a muscle, sprain an ankle or break a leg. In nature, you can die from a minor injury. The endurance predator laid up for two weeks with a sprained ankle might never come back. So the signals to your brain from strength training are loud and important: priority news. And they create growth—first in the signaling pathways themselves, blazing that direct trail through the forest of neural networks, and second in the muscles, tendons, ligaments and joints directly. With this growth comes a new integration between your brain and body. They have always been fused; we just forgot it. This is how you reconnect them. It's a literal, physical reconnection: nerve fibers you can see under the microscope, brain chemistry you can see on MRI scans, reaction time you can measure in the lab. It's skiing better, feeling stronger, feeling better.

It's also *not* falling down. As Chris mentioned, you're much more likely to fall as you get older unless you stay in great shape. This is a major public health issue, because you also fall harder and do more harm to yourself. C-6—*hiss* and, literally, *bump* in the night. Falls have been carefully studied, and it turns out you do not stumble any more often as you age; in other words, you catch your toe just as often as you did at twenty. But instead of easily recovering your balance, you're more likely to hit the pavement. There are two reasons for this. To begin with, you have let your proprioception slow down a critical bit. It takes a split second longer before your brain realizes you're falling, and in that split second momentum and gravity turn against you. The other point is that it takes strength to recover from a stumble. Your toe stops on the pavement, but your body keeps going, building up speed and momentum in a Newtonian drive

Steroids, Supplements and Snake Oil

We assume that you're one of the smart guys, but there's this pernicious human tendency to look for short cuts. Steroids add almost nothing to the average athlete; they just increase the water retention in muscles and make them bigger— but *not much stronger*. And among the probable side effects are impotence, prostate cancer, personality changes (not good ones), acne, hair loss and . . . impotence.

Supplements, the other instant miracle, have made absolutely no difference in any reliable scientific study. This goes for both strength training and Fountain of Youth type pills in general. There are rafts of badly done studies, funded by supplement makers, showing remarkable gains. But neither vitamins, nor supplements, nor hormones, nor special protein powders make any difference at all, no matter how deeply someone looks into your eyes while promising the opposite.

Our advice is to take a multivitamin daily, drink gallons of tap water, eat well and enjoy your body for what it is.

toward earth. By the time you move your leg, your entire body mass is moving forward and down with increasing speed. It's like jumping off a low wall. Your legs have to be strong enough to stop your momentum, or down you go.

Strength training gives you the power to fight gravity and stay on your feet. Even if you do take a fall, having strong reflexes and powerful muscles changes it from a head-on collision to a softer impact. Like the crumple zones in your car, your coordinated muscle action softens the blow. You will fall less if you are strong, and you will fall *better,* dramatically lowering your odds of serious injury.

Falls aside, strength training lowers your chance of injury with all forms of exercise—in large part by speeding up your proprioceptive reflexes, but also by strengthening your tendons, ligaments and joints. Tendons and ligaments are living tissue, but they grow more slowly as you get older. Pulling hard on a tendon strengthens the nerve connections and makes the tendon grow a bit farther into the bone, strengthening the attachment and rendering it more resistant to injury.

Find a Strength Sport

Weights are satisfying, perhaps even mildly addictive, but they're not fun for most people—which is why you need to see the payoff. My advice? Find a strength sport that you like, or learn to like one. Bicycling, skiing, tennis, squash, kayaking and canoeing are great ways to feel the measurable benefit of your time in the gym. Most guys find that strength training also markedly improves their golf game.

A Word About Arthritis

People with arthritis often see it as a barrier to strength training. But arthritis is not a contraindication. Quite the contrary. The combination of strong muscles and improved proprioception protects the joints from further damage and lets them heal. Most arthritis patients report about a 50 percent reduction in pain and limitation with several months of strength training; minor arthritis usually disappears entirely. All those aches and pain do make it trickier to get started, however, particularly if you have significant arthritis. If that describes you, talk to your doctor about having a physical therapist guide you in the initial stages of your weight-training program.

Once you're fit and pretty strong, you might try yoga. Whereas weights build specific muscle groups in isolation, yoga integrates strength and balance training. The rich sensory stimulation of using muscle groups in different combinations, and linking this with breathing, mind exercises and stretching, creates a more profound neurosensory and proprioceptive integration than Western exercise. *But beware:* The injury potential from yoga in our culture is quite high. You have to be reasonably fit to start yoga; after all, it was created by people who were *already* living a very physical life. Moreover, we have an aerobics class mentality that asks us to do more and better each day. If you do try yoga, think about starting with individual instruction for five sessions. It's expensive but well worth it, and if the instructor doesn't teach you how to listen to your body, find someone else. Group yoga classes, once you understand the basics, are among the best deals around, going for ten bucks in most places.

Whatever you decide to do, *do it*. Strength training is critical to the rest of your life, and you can start at any age. Sedentary, seventy-year-old men double their leg strength with three months of weight training. Sadly, men do strength training even less than aerobic exercise. Only 10 percent of Americans over sixty-five even *claim* to be doing *any* form of regular strength training.

That's appalling. It should be clear by now that everyone—certainly everyone over fifty—should be doing real strength training two days a week. You can do a quick routine in half an hour, or spend an hour or more if you get into it, but don't skip it. Aerobic exercise saves your life; strength training makes it worth living.

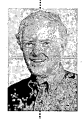

CHAPTER TWELVE

The Ugly Stick and Other Curiosities

isten, you've done a lot of heavy lifting in these first chapters. You've sat still for a lot of lecturing about exercise and some fairly heavy science from Harry. What do you say we relax for a couple of chapters and tell stories?

This chapter, for example, is a collection of bizarre little things that happen to people in the Next Third, which we thought you might be amused by. Actually, we thought it might be useful to know about them in advance so you won't be surprised. Or horrified. Things like forgetting the dog's name. Or going deaf. Or getting ugly. Oops. The idea is that, if you know this weird stuff is coming, you can just go to the door and let it in. Like a new pal. Go back to your chair and continue reading as if nothing had happened. Or, if you want to *do something*, go upstairs and take an ax to the hair that's suddenly growing out of your nose like a marijuana plant. Our purpose is merely to let you know that all this stuff is normal. And that normal is no longer your friend.

The Ugly Stick

Remember how, when you were a mean little kid, you made your nasty friends laugh by saying, "That Janey, man. She's so ugly, she must've been smacked with the *Ugly Stick*." Ho, ho, ho.

Well, there's an excellent chance that you'll get to atone for that bit of cruelty all those years ago. Tomorrow or the next day, you're likely to wake up in the morning and realize that you yourself have been tapped—maybe pretty hard—with the Ugly Stick. And you're going to know just how Janey felt. Once we're in our fifties or sixties, most of us go through this fundamental, deeply surprising change in how we look. Granted, the change only has to do with how *we look,* not *who we are,* but it's an odd experience and you may want to get in a crouch for it . . . get ready.

Suddenly, your skin gets weird, all over. If I take a pinch of muscle on my legs, the surface looks like crepe paper because the skin is old. My legs are pretty strong, but they *look* ridiculous. It happens to the skin on your pretty little face, too; how do you like that? You look different because the wrapper is getting sort of translucent. In fact, there's going to come a time when there are going to be little notches on your upper lip, as if your teeth were showing through. Ugh. And spots all over the place. And wattles all down your neck. I can toss my neck wattles over my shoulder when I go out in the morning, like a scarf. Nothing we do will prevent these things. They are normal.

I remember when it happened to me, my reaction was so comical it's hard to believe. I really thought there was a problem with my camera. All of a sudden, when a set of pictures came back from the developer, the ones of me were terrible. There was this dreadful distortion. My face had this *round* look. Like Frank Sinatra when he was old. There was way too much face, and not enough hair, so the ratios were all wrong. I thought about getting a new camera.

Good news and bad news. I did not need a new camera. But I was getting older, and I looked it. Not that I had been so wonderful-looking before, but this was much, much worse. And so sudden. I felt sad. Depressed, to tell you the truth. I wondered what I could do. The partial answer is . . . nothing. Some of this stuff is on the same biological time line as your declining maximum heart rate. Just happens. You're alive, aren't you? Quit whining.

But there are a few things you can do. All the exercise stuff in this book, for one. And the nutrition we're going to talk about next. And the alertness that invests the faces of people who are caught up in interesting affairs, which we talk about after that. All that helps tremendously. Old is old, but there's a huge difference between the look (and of course the feel) of a fit, engaged sixty- or seventy- or eighty-year-old . . . and some old loser who's fifty pounds overweight and waiting to die. So get in shape. Get involved in life. Get your muzzle out of the French fries. That will help a lot. As to the rest, get over it.

One of the nice things about being in good shape is that people go to the trouble of lying to you. I get it all the time: "What? You're seventy? Well, I never!" Sadly, that's nonsense. If there were money on it, they could guess my age to within a week. But in a sense, they're being honest. If you're fit, you do look better than the standard-issue old guy. Moral: Be a healthy, vibrant seventy or eighty and people will lie to you. And you'll believe them. You'll still get tapped with the Ugly Stick. But they won't hold you down and beat you like a dog.

Heroic Measures

Harry and I have a bias against heroic measures, like dyeing your hair or having a face-lift. But that's just a matter of personal preference. We don't happen to think there's anything wrong with looking like a healthy whatever-your-age. But both of us have close pals who do these things. And some of them, men and women, have had great pleasure in it. My beloved sister Petie had a massive face-lift at seventy-five. I called her a couple of weeks into the recovery to check how she was coming. "Well," she said, "I'm all black and blue and I'm still sixty pounds overweight. And I look *lovely*." She did, too. She looked like a girl for a while there—her face, anyhow—and it gave her tremendous pleasure.

A close friend had his eyes "done" and, somewhat to my surprise, it was a great success. So, do what you think best. Get a handle on the pain, though, and the expense and the risk; there's a fair amount of all of those. And don't undervalue the beauty of just being a good-looking old guy, because you're fit. And interested in your life.

Same goes for dyeing your hair. I think that guys who dye their hair look like guys who dye their hair. A variant of the poor creatures who fight baldness by combing their sparse hair over the tops of their heads. Take a close look at Donald Trump sometime; see what you think. I think it makes you look delusional. Of course, I happen to have my hair, so I may not be a good judge. If my hair suddenly starts to go—

or turns that stained-yellow-white that some guys get—I'll be at the hair dyer's in a heartbeat.

Whiten Your Teeth

Teeth are another matter. Nothing makes you look older and more pathetic than a scraggly mess of yellow teeth. By the time you're sixty, you've had a lot of nasty stuff in your mouth, and your teeth are probably stained an unpleasing Tuscan yellow. Well, fix 'em. I don't know why teeth are different from hair, but they are. Probably because I had those yellow teeth and not the bad hair. Anyhow, go to the dentist and tell him to dye 'em. Easy as pie and doesn't cost that much. And he won't give you a mouthful of bone-white ones that look fake. He'll just bring you back into the range of normal. Makes a difference in how you look and feel.

Just Say No to Yasir Arafat

You may be tempted, particularly when you're not going to the office every day, to forget about shaving. Don't. You may think "Bruce Willis!" but you may look "Yasir Arafat!" No matter what else is going on, get up in the morning, brush your teeth . . . and shave. Carefully. Patches of white whiskers, here and there, send a strong signal: "Old loser!"

I used to shave in the shower without a mirror. No more. Too easy to miss places. Now I shave in good light and go over and over the tough spots. It doesn't make me look young, but it does keep me from looking like an idiot.

While you're peeking in the mirror, get a pair of scissors and get those tusks of hair out of your nose. They grow like crazy all of a sudden, and you have to keep after them. Very important. Ears, too, if you can manage it. Be sure to go to a barber who's good about that. Unless you're a Hobbit, furry ears are a bad sign.

Adventures in the Skin Trade

Here's another interesting thing that happens in the Next Third. You get these little spots here and there. And they can kill you. Harry and I are not your mother. It is not our job to tell you to put on sunscreen and wear a hat when you go out to play. Or to go to the skin doc. But it is my job to tell stories. Here's one.

When I lived in the Rockies, everyone knew the air was thin, the sun was fierce and you had to be extra careful. Yap, yap, yap. How I *hate* to be lectured. So I *sometimes* wore sunscreen and even went to a dermatologist a couple of times. When I moved to New York, I eventually found a terrific one, whom you may remember from the first chapter. Cute as a button and smart as a whip. After some chitchat, she put on a little mask and took off half my nose. So I wouldn't die.

She was terrific, but that business of cutting off my nose was no fun. I am stubborn because I am old. But I wear hats now. And put on sun goop. And see my skin doc every four months. Don't want to do that nose thing again. Ever. (Did I mention that they "harvest" flesh from your ear to fill the hole they make? Yuck.)

Whether you start wearing goop or not—and it is more important now than ever—I beg you to go see a dermatologist. Old boys are stubborn about this, but listen: Skin cancer is mostly curable, and the cure is often a little zing with something cold. (Nose removal is reserved for the serious offender.) It is absolutely nuts for anyone over fifty not to get regular checkups.

Modern Dress
and Related Concepts

I am the last person on earth to talk about clothes, because I am clueless on the subject. Not as doomed as Harry, perhaps, but not good. Still, there are a couple of things to think about. I will keep my remarks brief. Consider the possibility of modern dress. You probably think you're in modern dress now, but there's an excellent chance that you're not . . . that your notion of how to dress was frozen the year you turned eighteen. When I went to my fiftieth high school reunion last spring, I was struck by the fact that all of us were dressed almost exactly alike. Soft-shouldered sport coats, button-down blue oxford cloth shirts, chinos or gray flannels. I thought we all looked nice. Hilary thought we looked Korean War.

At least consider the possibility of gingering yourself up a bit (there's an expression you haven't heard for a while) . . . gingering yourself up by trying something a little bit unfamiliar. A teeny bit modern. It doesn't matter much, but it may make you feel a little fresher, a little more adventurous. Go to a store you don't normally go to. Tog yourself out in black. Get some strange shoes. Personally, I have more or less decided *not* to have my ears pierced. Or my eyebrows. That's just not me. But I may eventually have some cosmetic surgery. And while I'm on the table, I may have the guy pierce my ears. And my eyebrows. But not my tongue, man. I'm not doing my tongue.

Older guys tend to care less about appearances. That's kind of appealing in a way. But appalling in another. Casual attire is one thing. Food all over yourself and your fly open is another. There's a real tendency to lose track of these things—the junk on the collar, the spots on the tie, the desperate need for a haircut. Don't go there. Get more rather than less interested in how you look, and you may come out even.

If you should have the good luck to get *really* old, my vote is that you become a fanatic about neatness and dress. It confuses people. Hilary and I have a wonderful pal, a guy in his late eighties, who's one of the most vibrant, interesting people either of us knows. And he is also one of the most meticulously togged-out people we know. Elegant. And it seems to be all of a piece with his vigor and charm. Personally, I am a New England frump. And Harry, of course, is much, much worse. That's not going to change. But I'm not going to let it get any worse if I can help it . . .

Grumpy Old Men

Here's some dark news. A lot of us get noticeably grumpier when we reach the Next Third. To my horror, I find that I, of all people, am particularly susceptible.

As you can perhaps tell by now, I have a generally sunny disposition. I was capable of being a bit stern in court, if absolutely necessary, but mostly I was pretty cheerful. Then, starting about five years ago, I noticed that I was snapping at Hilary. About the way she was driving. Or about her trying to tell me where to turn. Or taking forever to get dressed. Any damn thing. Then it spread to the traffic. I was snarling in traffic, blowing my horn in fury over this and that. Taking silly chances to prevent some stranger from getting ahead of me as we melded into one line. It was noticeable. It was awful. It was dumb.

And it was embarrassing. I have worked hard at avoiding the most obvious signs of aging, but here I was, walking across the street, giving the finger to some cabbie. I finally began to wonder, are there more outrages in the world, all of a sudden, or am I getting weird? The answer was, I was getting weird as if I had a huge sign on my chest saying "Grumpy old man!"

Okay, what do you do? My advice: Fight it like a steer. Think about it every time you want to rise up in righteous wrath at some poor taxi driver. Think about the strong possibility that the seething injustice you are about to crush is nothing. Even if it feels like the damnedest outrage you ever saw. Stop. Because you are probably making a fool of yourself. Write the letter but don't send it. Form the angry words in your head, but don't say them. *Do not trust your temper.* With these wise slogans in my head, I have done better. A teeny bit better. If you develop some good techniques, e-mail us. Do not become a grumpy old man if you can possibly help it. It is dreadful. But it is normal.

A Chow's Tail

Here's an engaging thing. A small percentage of guys, in their fifties or sixties . . . all of a sudden their penis when erect curls up like a chow's tail. All right, not like a chow's tail, but a distinct upward curl. Imagine . . . straight ahead and true for fifty years. And now it's looking, ever so slightly, up at the sky. You're terrified that you've "bent" it, in the course of doing something disgusting. What's going on?! Well, almost nothing, Harry says. For a certain number of guys, it just happens. Works fine, a bit curly is all. It's normal.

Sounding Funny

Once, when Mother was eighty and I was forty, we were driving along singing, as we often did. She had had a sweet voice all her life. Then that day her voice cracked, for no reason, in mid-song, and the notes went every which way, like a teenage boy. She started to laugh. Apparently, she used to tease her own mother about *her* voice breaking. And now, here she was, croaking away. Singing or talking, there comes a time when your voice changes and you sound like an old guy.

What to do? Mostly just laugh, like Mother. But if you happen to sing, you might do it a little more often. I know that most men my age—to say nothing of yours—don't sing at all, which is a shame. But the ones who do (including all the secret shower singers and solitary car singers) have a resource. Turns out a voice is one of those use-it-or-lose-it things. I sing like a lunatic when I'm in the shower or when I'm in the car. It's worked so far. I think.

Water

Here's a silly one: Drink more water. Surely one of the dullest pieces of advice in the book, but not stupid. One of the gadgets that goes to hell in the Next Third is the little thing that tells you you're thirsty. You don't feel thirsty, even though your body is crying out for water, which means old boys can have serious dehydration problems for no good reason at all. So, think about it, especially if you get serious about the exercise program. Dehydration can be awful for you. You may know this already, but one of the odd, if basic, facts I learned from Harry is that we have only five gallons of blood in our system. That's not a hell of a lot, when you consider all the stuff it has to do. Bring in the food. Take out the garbage. Carry all these amazingly sophisticated messages and chemicals. Flood your cells with good vibes. You want to keep your blood flowing smoothly.

Dehydration prevents blood from flowing smoothly. Your blood gets thick. It gets gummy and sludgy. Things start to go wrong in the outer provinces of your body, like your kidneys. And in the capital, too . . . your brain. Serious endurance athletes know firsthand how critical water is to performance. They are careful not to have too much at once (as in a garden, a constant trickle is better than a flood). And they make damn sure to have enough, which is a much more serious problem. They want to keep themselves hydrated above almost everything. You should, too. Because your thirst-signaling system may be on the blink.

Basic rule: Drink eight glasses of water a day (eight-ounce glasses, so that's sixty-four ounces a day). And add a quart for every hour you exercise. You may not feel like drinking that much. Make yourself.

How? Try this. Bang back one glass every morning, first thing, when you wake up. Maybe with that vitamin pill or your cholesterol pill or your baby aspirin. Same thing at night, when you go to bed. One more with each meal, that's obvious. Five down, three to go.

Okay, here's a particularly helpful one for you drinkers. The cocktail/hors d'oeuvres hour is a tricky part of the day. That hunger you feel may be a "false signal" for thirst. Just when you're tempted to have yourself lowered into the cheese dip, have a glass of water instead. You'll be surprised how often your "hunger" goes away. Another tip: Have a glass of water between every glass of wine or whatever it is you're drinking. You cannot hold as much booze as you used to, and this is a good way to slow yourself down. You've still got one more to go? You're a grown-up; think of something.

What?

At some point, your hearing starts to go. It's worst in crowd scenes . . . cocktail parties, restaurants and so on. It's annoying to you and infuriating to others. The greater risk, however, is that you will get isolated in your deafness just at a time when you ought to be struggling most to stay social. I'm not there yet (close, but not yet), but it seems to me that the guys who do best are the ones who go ahead and get the hearing aid, no matter how big and clumsy it feels (and they're not anymore) . . . no matter how stigmatizing they think it is (that's silly). My hearing doc tells me to wait until I really need one, but I am not going to wait too long. I want to get used to it and get into it, while I'm still a teeny bit flexible. And before the notion of *not* hearing what's going on around me starts to feel appealing. Don't get isolated.

Slow Down.
Look Both Ways. Repeat.

Remember all my tiresome stories about falling down for no reason? I know it won't happen to you because of the weights you've started to lift, but keep that problem in mind, just in case. And bear in mind that the process that makes you fall down in the street is also at work when you drive a car or ski or bike. Older people have more accidents. Including, to my horror, me. Try this: I was backing up to turn around in my own flat, open driveway. Degree of difficulty: 1.0. I am a good driver, and I was backing up pretty crisply. And I backed hard into my very own car, which was sitting in the driveway in plain sight. Damage: $3,000. Hilary loved the call to the insurance company: "Hi. This is Chris Crowley, your insured . . . blah blah blah. Say . . . uh, does my insurance cover my, uh, driving into my own car?"

What's going on in these situations, as you know, is that your proprioception is tailing off. And it's dangerous. You recognize it in others, but you may not recognize it in yourself, because the very idea seems preposterous. Which it is. But it happens just the same. Watch for it, and if you find yourself having some falls or some minor driving mishaps, slow down, because the consequences are so very serious. Don't be ashamed, don't be embarrassed . . . just slow down a little. And look around a bit more than usual. The stakes are very high, and your margin of error is narrower. I will almost never say this, but "act your age."

That advice applies to skiing, boating, horseback riding . . . you name it. Your sense of where you are and your control of your own body are both going south. I hope you are fighting it with weights and cross-training, because that really works, but it does not make you bulletproof.

For an ongoing report on these and other curiosities—and if you have any for us—see our Web site, *www.younger nextyear.com.*

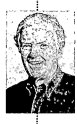

CHAPTER THIRTEEN

Chasing the Iron Bunny

The subject of this chapter, personal economy, could have been tucked neatly into "The Ugly Stick," along with the other curiosities of aging and retirement, but we thought it was so important that it should have its own short space. Harry even gave it its own rule. Think of this as a weird little peppermint to clear your palate before we turn to the chapters on eating. Or a magic pill to prevent half the anxiety and pain of retirement. Whatever your age, you can't start thinking about this business too soon.

There's one change that hits in retirement that you cannot duck and that you must prepare for as early as possible: *There's less dough.* It's not as awful as you think, unless you don't deal with it. In which case it will kill you dead. And all our other happy talk about working out and being functionally younger and everything else won't make a bit of difference. Because you will be dead of anxiety. So Harry's Fourth

Rule goes like this: *Spend less than you make.* Seems obvious, doesn't it? And yet there are ever so many men, at all income levels, who get messed up by failing to follow it, especially in retirement.

People go into a fugue state on this stuff. They go off to a land of dreamy dreams and assume it will somehow take care of itself. Well, it won't. It will take care of you. And your darling wife. And your little dog, Toto. You will all be deep out of luck unless you force yourself to look this one in the eye and plan a little. If you don't, when the fog lifts, you may be on the rocks. You do not want to be swimming away from the wreckage at seventy.

Having a plan, even if it's imperfect, will make you much better off. And you'll be better off still if you can get over the notion that dough and material stuff are as important as you think they are. You can live perfectly happily on much less if you quit chasing the iron bunny of material and status and things that you don't really want or need.

We are not financial advisers, for sure, but we ask you to sit down right now and make a realistic estimate of how much income per year you're going to have in retirement. Next, unless your income is inflation-protected, adjust it downward. Then assume things will be a bit worse and cut it 5 percent more. You may also want to take a hard look at some of your prospective sources of income, calculate coldly just how reliable they are and make appropriate adjustments. Okay, that's your annual income. Teeny, isn't it? Now come up with a lifestyle and plan—a modest house in a less expensive town, perhaps—that will let you live on less than that. And you will be safe and happy from then on. No matter how small the house or how tight the lifestyle, it will be *joyous* when contrasted with the eventual lifestyle of guys who do not go through this analysis.

If you are borderline honest with yourself, you will probably see that you'll be living on a small fraction of your earnings peak. Say, two-thirds or a half. Maybe even a quarter, which is where I wound up. Depending on various things, that can be a painful difference.

As ever, there's good news and bad news. The good news first: Above the poverty level, there is no correlation between money and happiness. Elaborate surveys say this is so. Think about it. You've been struggling for more dough all your life, and there is no correlation between money and happiness. How can that be? I don't know, but apparently it's true.

So what's the bad news? *Deciding* to live on less is way, way hard. We think we *are* what we own. Or drive. Or eat. Or wear. We are material and status junkies. And like all junkies, we are absolutely convinced that we gotta have it. Gotta have money/status/power. We've been trained to chase the iron bunny, like the greyhounds at the racetrack, and we cannot get over it. We have so much invested in what we make . . . how many empty rooms we have in the house . . . how many seconds from zero to sixty in the gas piggy . . . how big the office. We've been persuaded that we are what we make. The firm, the practice, the corporation held money out to us and focused all our attention on it. And like dopes, we bought it. The iron bunny, my man, and we barked and wagged our tails and ran like lunatics. Not for the nourishment, God knows, but because *that was the game.*

It's not hard to quit eating iron rabbits. But it's very hard not to *want* to eat iron rabbits. You have to persuade yourself that *that* game is over. Never mind whether or not it was a good game or how terrific you were at it . . . it's over. Time to quit playing and come inside. Come inside your income. Try to do it early. As with smoking, you can recover. It takes time and earlier is better, but do it. Get over the game or it will kill you, just as sure as God made little tin cups. Some of the most wretched old people out there are some of the smartest and, formerly, the most successful. But they could not learn this simple truth. They thought the old rule was so fundamental that they'd be better off as alcoholics, say, than guys in smaller houses or older cars. Until it was too late.

It's entirely possible that you are not going to retire after all. You may work forever. But you have to plan for that prospect, too. Figure out what you *can* do. Where you can do it, and so on. Think about connections . . . retraining . . . whatever makes sense. But do it early and do it with a touch of realism. The best plan for many is some combination of postretirement work and a much simpler lifestyle. Not a bad prospect at all; a lot of people find that full retirement is overrated. But it does take planning. Do it now.

The difficulties of turning your back on old spending levels run a lot deeper than just living within your means. What we're really talking about here is stepping out of the endless struggle for status in the pack that ran our lives for the last forty years. That's the subject of some serious talk in the final chapters of the book, and it involves some very serious and difficult issues. Briefly, it goes like this. From the time you were a teenager, you were obsessed—and encouraged to be obsessed—with your status in a particular pack. Your clique in high school . . . your company or law firm in adulthood . . . your country club . . . your bowling league. That particular game, whatever it was worth, is over for you. Live within your means and forget how it looks to the rest of the pack. They're over at the dump now, anyway, sniffing for fresh garbage. Look after yourself. On your own terms. And find a new pack.

If you're having trouble with this, go to a financial adviser . . . it's money well spent. (Get a stand-alone adviser, not one who makes his money getting you to buy this and that financial product.) Or read one of the good books on the subject. A fun one that I found useful is *The Millionaire Next Door.* (Turns out that the guys who really amass some dough never did buy into the notion that spending marks success. They held on to their dough and eventually became rich.) There are lots of others.

What Harry and I can do is remind you of some home truths that have special relevance in the Next Third. For example, The Dickens Truth: Income $100/expenses $99 equals happiness. Income $100/expenses $101 equals misery. Dickens did it in pounds sterling, but it works in all currencies. The other rule: Money cannot buy happiness, but spending more than you have can put your head in the toilet. Which your creditors will dutifully flush.

As that financial adviser will tell you, and as we said before, step one is to figure out just how much you can expect on a *conservative basis* to have per year for the next thirty years. (Remember, you're going to live a long, long time.) A real number. Then take a shy peek at your expenses and your lifestyle. Then apply the ax.

It looks as if it will be terribly painful, but please remember: Contrary to what we're taught in all the ads, it is not your winkie you are carving down to size, it's just the stuff you eat and hang on the walls. Relax. This won't hurt that much. Unless you don't do it. Spend less than you make . . . much less. Get that problem off the table. There's not much that you're "too old for," but you're too old for this nonsense.

A good idea: Decide, with your partner, just which of you is best at managing money and let that person do it, regardless of who made it. Or do it together. Make a plan . . . write stuff down. Take it seriously. Anxiety is bad for old boys. Very bad.

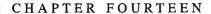

Don't You Lose a Goddamn Pound!

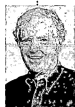

arry and I are serenely aware that an $88 billion check is waiting for the guy who comes up with the next blockbuster diet book that says *his* gimmick really *does* work and will make you lose fifty pounds in two weeks and keep it off for the rest of your life. Because there are 200 million chubby Americans who are panting to believe it. Well, tough. It's not true. And we're not going to take your money. The dreary, persistent fact is that diets don't work; 95 percent of them fail, which is why setting weight loss as a goal is generally a bum idea. The almost certain failure can infect your attitude toward fitness, while the yo-yoing up and down actually makes you gain weight. So don't diet. That's the headline. Our advice is, basically, forget about it. But exercise six days a week and follow Harry's Fifth Rule. Which is: *Quit eating crap!*

Now the small print. Will there come a time, way down the road, when you lose a pound or two on this regimen? Just for fun? Not dieting? Yeah, that could happen. You might lose forty, as a matter of fact, the way I did. There's a pretty good chance of it, to tell you the truth. If you do, just send us the $88 billion when you have a moment. But not now, please. We won't take it. The thing to do now is *get in shape*. Go back and read the first few chapters and start to exercise! Because exercise does work, whether or not you're fat as a walrus. It is always the first step, the bit of magic, as I said in the beginning, that changes everything. So focus on that, quit eating crap and forget about weight loss.

Harry's Fifth Rule may seem a little vague to you, but you'd be surprised at how much you know intuitively right now. I urge you to sit down, this second, and make a list of all the mountains of garbage you're eating that you *know* you should quit eating altogether. I bet you get it 85 percent right *before* you read our two nutrition chapters. (Hint to get you started: French fries. Almost all fast food. Processed snacks with names that end with the letter "O.")

Exercising and not eating crap is not a diet, and you won't fail at it. If you don't lose weight, you will still be radically better off and functionally younger. If you lose weight, it's a bonus.

The God That Lied

Dieting is the False God of the last thirty years. The whole country has been on an extraordinarily expensive series of diets for at least that long. We have spent billions on them. Enough to send every kid in Texas and Massachusetts to law school and still have enough dough left over to fund class actions against every fast-food chain in the nation. And what did we get for our money? We gained forty pounds apiece, a handful of guys got rich and the rest of us got fat. Not a good use of our dough. Or our time. In fact, it was a ridiculous, shaming waste. So maybe we should cut it out.

As you might expect of a False God, the various bibles of dieting are not very reliable or consistent. The rich zealots who preach the True Faith cannot begin to agree on the sacred texts. I am not just talking about the weird, head-on conflict between Pritikin-Ornish (low fat, low fun) and Atkins (high fat, high fun . . . until recently, when poor Dr. Atkins died and his successors-in-interest backed off a bit from the eat-steak-till-you-drop claims). I am talking about the mainstream, center-of-the-road health establishment. Like the American Heart Association and the United States Department of Agriculture (USDA).

Remember the USDA health pyramid? And the magic of "carbo-loading"? Especially in the early 1990s, pasta was king, and rice and potatoes weren't far behind. In 1992, when many of us were looking for responsible guidance, the USDA created its new Food Guide Pyramid, which looked like this:

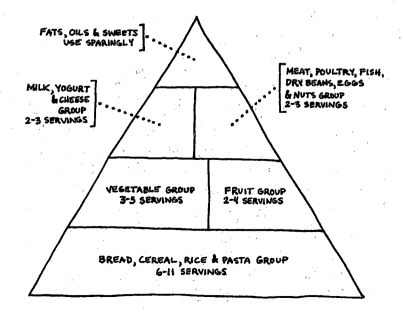

Look familiar? Of course it does. It's still on every box of Wheat Thins and Triscuits in the country. Yum, yum. Cracker makers love it. And bakers. And purveyors of French fries.

The trouble is, virtually everybody else now agrees that it is almost totally wrong. Less than nine years later, Dr. Walter C. Willett, chairman of the Department of Nutrition at the Harvard School of Public Health, published a pyramid in his *Eat, Drink, and Be Healthy: The Harvard Medical School Guide to Healthy Eating*. It looked like this:

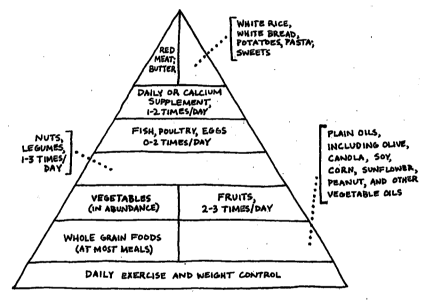

Oops! Take a close look. These lads cannot both be right. And it looks today as if the USDA was and is wrong. Think what a wild change that is, in just nine short years. Look at the carbs. From being among the foods you were supposed to eat most, white bread, white rice and pasta are now among the foods you're supposed to eat least. That's odd, isn't it? Isn't there a scientific community out there that's supposed to keep track of this stuff? And how about fat? In the old USDA pyramid, all fats are near-taboo. Now the good fats (olive oil and the like) are listed as among the best things you can eat.

So the question arises: Does anyone here know what he's talking about? Well, yes and no. On the "no" side, most diets are utterly unproven scientifically or medically. Not because their proponents are all dopes or charlatans, although there are certainly some of those. And neither is it some massive conspiracy of corporate farmers, fast-food restaurants, lobbyists and rotten politicians that's responsible, although they play a real part. Rather, as Harry points out, there simply is not a lot of good science on specific foods available.

The real difficulty is that every bite of food you take is a hugely complex blend of thousands and thousands of chemicals that interact in millions of important ways with different parts of your body. No one has taken the deep dive into the biology and chemistry to see what happens. Indeed, no one knows if it's possible to do so. So it's no surprise that no one has begun to devise tests to evaluate individual foods.

Harry puts the problem in an interesting light. He talks about President Kennedy's decision in 1961 to spend a fortune and put a man on the moon within the decade. Which we did. But, Harry says, if Abraham Lincoln had said that and spent the same amount of money, nothing would have happened. Same thing for Teddy Roosevelt. Or FDR. You cannot go to the moon with steam engines; the fundamental science has to be in place. That would be the problem today if a theoretical president decided to "solve" the national obesity problem with a breakthrough pill or diet or whatever it took. You could spend the dough, but you wouldn't get there, because the core science does not exist.

Which is not to say that we have to sit here and eat pizza and French fries for two hundred years while the scientists beaver away. There are, for example, broad population studies that show that the diet historically followed by the good people of Okinawa was healthy. The Okinawans were the longest-lived people on earth until they shifted to a Western diet. Personally, I take greater comfort in the fact that the Mediterranean diet also gets high marks. I find it a little more accessible. Lots of yummy vegetables, olive oil, some meat and a sufficiency of red wine . . . I'm there.

It may occur to you that these are mighty "broad brush" evaluations . . . deciding that a whole country or all of southern Europe is eating "good" food. Sounds a little rough, doesn't it? In fairness to the nutrition community, narrower, more *scientific* population studies are very hard to conduct. Ideally, they would involve large numbers of normal people and last for, oh, ten years, testing this and that food. Broccoli, say. Well, who in the world is going to eat broccoli for ten years and keep a record of it? And who is going to volunteer to be in the control group that has to eat rat poison *with* their broccoli? So it is slow work. But we know enough to set out a few rules.

Yes, Virginia, Calories Do Count

Once-popular books to the contrary notwithstanding, calories do count. They are, ultimately, the only things that count. So one can say, with utter confidence, that the secret behind getting fat is eating more calories than you burn. Surprise. As far as getting fat is concerned—as opposed to getting heart attacks and cancer and whatnot—it doesn't much matter what kind of calories they are. For obesity, 100 calories of spinach is no better and no worse than 100 calories of French fries. It's the old gag about which is heavier, a ton of feathers or a ton of lead? Same deal here: Calories are calories.

Well, not exactly the same deal. Some foods take a certain amount of energy just to digest. Those yummy fibers, for example. All that bran. (They taste it, too, don't they?) If you can hack it, it makes sense to eat more of those, because they fill you up and keep you filled while they work their way endlessly through your digestive system. They contain some good health stuff, too.

Start to get an idea in your head of what an ideal level of calorie consumption should be for you. It's a sad fact that your base metabolism, the rate at which you burn calories automatically, without exercise, goes down steadily as you age. That—and the sedentary habits of older people in our society—is where that gut comes from after forty. Or fifty. A normal American in his fifties or sixties has to get his caloric intake down to roughly 1,500 calories to lose weight. Up to 2,000 a day is maintenance. Get an idea of how many calories you're taking in during a day. Get one of those little books and look up a few of the things that you eat most often. It's easier than you think, because all of us eat in a relatively narrow band. And you don't have to worry much about the fruits and vegetables and fish, because they are so low-calorie that they're almost free. Just keep track of the booze, the carbs, the meat and the sugars. You don't have to be precise, but have an idea of your caloric intake. That is, after all, where all the weight comes from. All the triumphs and all the failures. Calories in . . . calories out.

Which raises the important but depressing issue of portion control. We've gone nuts, in this country, with the size of our portions. Food purveyors push supersizes and all-you-can-eat menus because it doesn't cost the fast-food places much to double your portion. It costs you quite a lot. Do not clean your plate. Do not eat like a pig and call it virtue.

Short-Cycle Hunger Spikes

Another important point, as Harry is about to tell you, is that some foods—especially carbs and sugars—spike short, intense cycles of renewed hunger. You feel hungrier, sooner, after a plate of French fries than after a bowl of spinach. Because almost no one can resist those hunger spikes, it makes plenty of sense to limit—not eliminate—carbs and simple sugars. Personally, when it comes to carbs, I don't have to wait for the hunger spike. I can eat them until I drop. Eat the whole loaf of French bread and butter, before the menus are passed out. Eat the entire bucket of popcorn. The whole bowl of pasta. I am never tempted to eat spinach or codfish like that. Sadly.

But even if you have more willpower than I do, you should sharply limit your consumption of white bread, white rice, pasta, potatoes and sweets. They are at the tippety-top of the new pyramid, and they belong there. Incidentally, French fries, which I adore with all my heart, deserve their own circle in hell. They should be the flagpole on the top of the pyramid. They start as potatoes, so they're carbs at the core. Then they're routinely cooked in saturated fats, which makes them much, much worse. If there is evil in the universe, it is made manifest in the design of the French fry, which tastes so heavenly and is in fact the devil's own food.

Which brings me to those things that are so awful for you that they should be banned altogether—a list that is going to vary from person to person. My personal diet guru, the wise Stephen Gullo, has great advice about how to deal with food we know is rotten for us but love: Drop it altogether. His favorite quote to me was "For those who are given to excess, abstinence is easier than moderation."—John Drybred. Best nutrition advice I ever got. For me, as you may have guessed, that means no more French fries. Maybe for you, too. And having no bread is way easier than a little bit. I have lapses, but not so many. And I know enough to feel guilty!

Quit Eating Fast Food

The science of nutrition is imperfect, and our understanding is weak—but not so weak that we do not know that the brightly lit fast-food signs are guiding us to a dark place. I don't want to spend the rest of my life in court, so let's just look at the new food pyramid, then at the McDonald's menu, and let some things speak for themselves. (Burger King or a host of others would do as well.) Remember, before we begin: Calories count. Red meat, white bread, potatoes, sugar and saturated fat are bad. Okay, McDonald's . . . what have we got under the golden glow?

Hilary and I just walked over to the McDonald's on our corner to see what's cooking. It's across from a public high school for which it serves as commissary and hangout; it's jammed with kids. Good news and bad news, again. The good news is plastered all over the windows out front. Big posters pushing "McDonald's Real Life Choices." Happy talk of lunches and dinners for under 400 calories, breakfasts under 300. Hooray for McDonald's . . . or for their lawyers. This place is a garden of dietary responsibility and care for these kids who almost live there. What an about-face.

Let's go inside. More great news: Super Size Fries and Super Size Cokes are still listed on the big menu board, but the price slots are empty. That's because they don't sell them anymore. Nope, these folks *will not sell you* a supersize Coke (410 calories) or a supersize order of fries (610 calories). They're just not that kind of girl now. Well, not *exactly* that kind of girl. Turns out they will sell you a large order of fries, which is a whopping 10 percent smaller (540 calories) and a large Coke, which is about 25 percent smaller (310 calories). Let's see what else is going on.

Oh, here's today's only special. It's $5.39 for a Big Mac (the reason we're all here), a medium side of fries and a medium Coke. And a "free music download from Sony Connect." This is the hot item. That's funny—there's no indication of how many calories this meal has. You have to go around the corner to an enormous chart with lots of small print to get that.

Okay, I've read the small print. The special contains 1,430 calories. Gee, that's way more than three times the calories in the meals touted in the window . . . and they forgot to tell us? Do you remember the term "bait and switch"? Probably not. Anyhow, 1,430 calories are almost enough to take a grown man through a full day. And almost all of them are rotten for you. The Big Mac has 600 calories, 300 of them from fat. The fries are 520 calories, 230 from fat; the Coke is 310 calories, all of them from sugar or corn syrup. That's the real "real life choice" at McDonald's. My take is as follows. The good news is in the window, and the bad news is going down the gullets of those kids (and grown men who act as if they don't know better). My modest suggestion? *Quit eating fast food! Do not go in the door!* True, some of these places are getting better, but basically they are gardens of evil. You don't go to a house of ill repute for conversation, and you don't go to a fast-food place for salad! Quit kidding yourself.

A last word on traditional fast-food places. Think of how they resemble those hideous factory farms where they make some of the slop we eat. Think of the vast piggeries down in North Carolina, where they force-feed millions of pigs that never step out of their narrow, agonizing pens from the day they're born to the day they're slaughtered. The "farms" that are poisoning the groundwater for miles around. Doubtless I am over the top, but I think of fast-food places as factory farms for people. We go there by the millions, like hogs to slaughter, and eat ourselves stupid, as if it were our jobs to become obese. Just like those poor piggies in North Carolina. All to make the fast-food people rich, regardless of the horror for us. Well, the hell with that. Don't go. And for God's sake, don't let these people set up shop in your schools. Don't *teach* your own precious kids to eat crap.

Look at the Pyramid; Look at the Label

Now that you know the black-letter rules, how do you comply with them? Well, you get several shots at not eating crap: in the food market, when you buy things; in your home, when you decide what to cook; and at the table, when you decide what and how much to put in your greedy mowzer. At each of those stages, try to think just a little bit about what's good for you and what's rotten. And try to act like a grown-up.

You also get three choices with restaurants. One, you do not have to go to places that specialize in food that's horrible for you. Two, in the restaurant, you can order things that are good for you (and ask the waiter to take the bread away, immediately). Three, once the damn stuff is on your plate, you don't actually have to eat it. Three strikes, my man. Think about each one.

In addition, you should take grateful advantage of food labeling. Lord knows how it happened, in this militantly capitalistic/laissez-faire nation, but labeling is required by law, and it's pretty good. The type is small, but the information is huge. Learn to look at the label. Learn not to eat much with saturated fat in it. And try to stay away completely from the real killers, the trans fats. (The reference is to "partially hydrogenated oils" of one kind or another on the label.) And stay away from foods with lots of calories. Or lots of carbs. Easy-peasy. Eventually, looking at labels becomes kind of fun. You are often surprised to find really tasty stuff that is superlight on calories. You are even more often stunned to see how many calories and carbs some of your oldest and best-loved friends have been packing all these years. I pick up a box of pasta from time to time to see if it's *still* true that this pleasant little package contains, say, a thousand calories. I used to empty those packages into my tummy and thought I was doing myself a favor. Not so. *Read the label!*

Anyhow, cruise the shelves and look for food that tastes good, that's made of good stuff and doesn't have that many calories. It's a scavenger hunt. Be super careful to check the portion size that goes with the calorie number. They are little cheats. On a can of soup, for instance, you'll find a reasonable calorie number—only to discover that the little can allegedly holds seventeen servings. It's an insidious species of lying. There's talk about fixing it. Be careful anyway.

It Is Possible to Eat Fish

You're a guy, right? And not completely nuts about change? So, at this late stage in the proceedings, how can anyone expect you to make fundamental alterations in your *diet,* for heaven's sake? I can only say, you'd be surprised. When I got on this kick, I'd been eating crap, happily, eagerly, compulsively, for sixty years. Most of my life, I had gotten away with it. Starting at about fifty, my luck ran out, and I went from 155 pounds to 207. Not nice. Eventually I got back to about 170, which was a joy. I'm about 180 now, which I can live with. But along the way I learned some things. The most striking example: I have always hated fish. *Hated* it. Ate it, under protest, twice a year. I kept being told, however, how great it was for you and what a key it was to weight loss and weight control. With reluctance bordering on horror, I tried it again. Never mind the details, but I now eat fish five nights a week. And I do it for pleasure. And those rye crisp crackers that are made out of cardboard and twigs and taste horrible? I now eat them like peanuts. *Love 'em.* And I never eat the popular crackers that were the beloved staples of my youth and middle age. By the way, here's a nice labeling story. There is now a version of Wheat Thins that bears the breathless logo "New Low Fat!" Take a peek at the nutrition label. The old, bad Wheat Thins were 150 calories a portion. The new ones, 130 calories a portion. No wonder these guys were breathless.

Lose Forty Pounds

Okay, time for a little shift in emphasis. Maybe it would not be such a bad idea, after all, if you lost forty pounds or whatever it would take to get back to your true weight. No rush. And no diet. It will just take care of itself because once you start exercising seriously, you'll see yourself differently and you'll start to feel a little odd being overweight. You probably feel a little odd now, but that's not what I mean. Once you get in shape and get into the business of working out, pushing yourself a little, it will start to seem, oh, *inappropriate* to be overweight. I don't know quite how, but it just happens. Then, whether gradually or in a plunge, your weight starts to drop. You really could lose forty pounds. Without going nuts and without going on a diet. Sort of.

I heard a lovely story recently about a friend's father. This guy retired at sixty-five and moved to Key West. A Navy officer in World War II, he had some pals down there, liked to golf and all that. He weighed 210 pounds when he retired. He smoked, and he drank a bottle of red wine every day, all by himself. But pretty soon he noticed that a number of his old buddies were dying, and he thought he'd skip that for a while. He started swimming, and he started going to the gym and doing weights and working with a trainer. He really got into it and loved it. Without dieting or going into any particular program, he steadily got his weight down. In a couple of years, he weighed 155, his weight in college. He worked out five or six days a week and eventually got into tae kwon do. At the age of eighty-two, he got his first-degree black belt. At eighty-six, he got his second-degree black belt. He died last fall at the age of ninety-one. At the time, he still weighed 155 pounds. He was still tight with some of his old Navy pals. And he still drank a bottle of red wine, every day, which we think is way too much. But his life was good.

We sure don't guarantee results like that, and we urge you not to obsess about them, but it could happen. I almost did it, and I am resolutely greedy and self-indulgent, as you know by now. I confess that I actually did some dieting, which we do not recommend, but the essence of it was exercise and a change of self-image.

Have a Picture of Yourself in Mind

A critical trick is to have the right picture of yourself in your head. Exercise makes that much easier. Working out, you automatically have the picture of your young self in your head. It feels natural to get rid of the excess that just doesn't *belong* there . . . like putting down a package you've been carrying for too long.

Incidentally, whole societies, whole countries, find obesity so profoundly at odds with the picture they have of themselves that it just doesn't happen. Not because of different genes or even different food, but because it's just out of the question. Think of how many fat Japanese people you know. Or Frenchmen, come to that. In those countries, it isn't done. Make obesity *your* taboo. Draw a picture in your head—of you on that bike or in the hills or on the boat— so strong and sharp and clear that being a big fat guy is *just out of the question.* Sound a little mystical? Far-fetched? Try it. Once you've become younger, sometime next year, you'll want to look it, too. And you may.

Exercise and Weight

Few of us are going to lose weight directly by exercising, because it takes far too much exercise to burn off significant fat. Olympic endurance athletes burn 4,000 to 6,000 calories a day, but they're working out like maniacs four, five and six hours a day, every day. You're not going to do that. You'll actively burn off a lot more calories than a sedentary man, but not enough for major weight loss. Still, by building up your muscle mass over time, you do help yourself significantly. Whether or not you're being active, muscles require a lot more food, a lot more energy, just for maintenance, than does fat. More mitochondria burning away, night and day, whether you're doing anything or not. So, once you get in shape, you're constantly burning more energy, even when you're not working out.

Everyone burns some 60 percent of the calories taken in just sitting around, on idle. That percentage goes up for those who exercise and have a greater lean muscle mass. Harry says you can increase your basal metabolism by 50 percent with rigorous exercise. That is huge.

The other way exercise works, of course, is that it really helps your self-image. Take a look around the gym. You'll see a few fat people, and it's entirely possible to pursue a heavy exercise regimen when you're very heavy yourself. I've done it. But it's not common. Look around a yoga class and you'll see what I mean. Maybe they're all self-selected and they looked like that the day they walked in, but I doubt it. I think that, like me . . . like that guy in Key West . . . like a lot of people I talk to in gyms around the country . . . they just lost the weight somehow, once they got in shape, once they got that new picture in their heads. I remember sitting on my bike in spinning class those first months. The rooms are always mirrored, as you know, and I could not take my eyes off myself. I found myself staring, hypnotically, obsessively, at the folds around my gut. I didn't want to lug the flab around, now that I was doing all this vigorous stuff.

But again, we're talking about being younger—and thinner—next year. And the year after that. We're talking about a fundamentally different lifestyle, and it will take a while to kick in. That's all right; you're going to live a long time. So exercise hard and get interested in life. Thin will take care of itself.

CHAPTER FIFTEEN

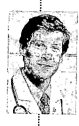

The Biology of Nutrition: Thinner Next Year

The message from thousands of studies, over decades of medical research, is clear: *Never go on a diet again.* The only way to lose weight is to embark on a program of steady, vigorous exercise, avoiding the worst foods being thrust upon you in our national diet and eating less of everything. I wish that were not true, but it is. This is not a diet chapter; it's a nutrition chapter. So, as Chris already told you, quit eating crap. Here's why.

As you might expect, we'll be going back to Darwin and how your Darwinian body reacts to various foods. This way, you'll understand what we mean when we urge you not to go into "famine mode," which will make you fat. And you'll understand why we urge you to avoid the junk foods that make you ravenous and are inflammatory for your cells.

The first and most basic point is that your Darwinian body does not know what to make of excess. It does not know what to do in the face of steady doses of too much food. It was not designed for *over*abundance or idleness, and it reacts in crazy ways. It reacts as if they were signals of famine.

Back in nature, every calorie was precious, so our early ancestors developed very specific—and very successful—ways to handle predictable swings in the food supply. There are seasonal variations in the fat content of our bodies that are as old as time. Winter, the dry season, migration: we have faced episodic famine since the beginnings of life. Our bodies respond by storing up fat and cutting down radically on the use of energy. This biology is locked deep in our bodies—and in the bodies of every other animal on the planet.

You might think—from our own reaction to plenty—that all animals would pack away as much fat as possible whenever there was extra food at hand, but that's not true. Animals put on or drop fat in response to more subtly perceived need. Fawns, for example, stop growing in October and start storing the calories they eat as fat to survive the winter, regardless of how big they are or how much food there is. In the spring, they start to use the calories to grow again, to build bone and muscle, *and they don't get fat* no matter how much food there is. They grow bigger if there's more food, but they don't store fat. Humpback whales store massive amounts of fat as they feed in their summer grounds in the North Atlantic and then, using their blubber as fuel, migrate thousands of miles to their calving grounds near the equator. They do not eat at all for six months, surviving by using every calorie of stored fat to its maximum potential. Migrating birds, feeding on shrimp in Chesapeake Bay in the fall, double their fat reserves in less than a week and then fly nonstop to Africa, but in the spring, when there is even more food, they grow muscle and bone, and the females lay eggs. They don't get fat.

The fundamental reaction to *springtime* for most animals is to invest extra calories in lean muscle and growth. To grow stronger and bigger, not fatter, even when there is plenty of food around. For males, it's the time to grow new tissue, like muscles, bones and sinew: partly to hunt, but also to compete for mates. For females, it's all of this, but it's also time to invest every extra scrap of energy in pregnancy. Women do store some fat to prepare for pregnancy, but not a lot, and it's not the same thing as obesity. There is a natural time to become fat, but it's heading into winter, not springtime. Fit-and-lean is the natural reaction to springtime. Game abounds, you are a healthy predator, and you surely do not want to burden yourself with an extra thirty pounds of fat.

But in times of incipient famine, that is exactly what you would want to do—like a bear going into hibernation or a deer on the edge of winter. So what are the signs of famine for humans? For us, the primary signal of famine was sedentary life. In the absence of food to hunt, we just sat around, conserving energy in that slow race with death. It's the sitting around that your body hears. Lock that image in your head. Your body reads idleness as a sign that you are starving to death as slowly as possible, *no matter how much you eat.*

Exercise Against Decay

The signals of approaching famine may differ between humans and other animals, but the biology of our reactions is essentially identical. It is the biology of decay. As you know by now, this whole book has one core message—either you grow or you decay. And sure enough, that's the essence of the biology of nutrition as well. Put simply, the chemistry behind obesity involves decay. Shutting down every system you possibly can so that you can survive winter, drought or famine. The fact that there *is* enough to eat today, or even vast excess, doesn't change this. If you are sedentary, your body reads the bacon cheeseburger as the carcass of the animal that starved to death just before you—your last-gasp chance to gorge. And here's an interesting thing. This biological response is turned on by our old friend C-6 and turned off by the C-10 of exercise. Scientists have known this for only a few years, but it makes perfect sense. C-6 and C-10 are, after all, the fundamental messengers of growth and decay.

That is why the single best thing you can do to stay or reverse obesity is to be physically active—to exercise consistently enough to send those springtime signals every day. The point of exercise is *not* to "burn off" calories, but rather to tell every part of your body to grow, to invest in building new tissue, and to run at a higher metabolic rate all day and all night long. Burning those extra calories is what does the job, even while you sleep. Losing weight will take some time, but it will occur. Ultimately, you will have to eat less, because you can overwhelm the most active metabolism with sheer caloric volume, but this becomes easier as you get in shape. Your body doesn't want the excess fuel, and your self-image changes, automatically and unconsciously, over a few months or a year. So keep portion control in the back of your mind. Let it percolate through your sense of self, and someday you'll find yourself feeling full after the appetizer and enjoying a salad for lunch. Until then, just focus on cutting out the stuff that's killing you.

Quit Eating Starch: The White Foods

One of the foods that are killing you is starch (refined carbohydrates), which means the current buzz about bad carbohydrates is basically correct. (How refreshing to have a major food fad turn out to make some sense.) Bad carbs are the white foods—potatoes, white rice, and pretty much everything made with refined flour. The good carbohydrates are the ones found in nature—in fruits, vegetables and whole grains, which have relatively few calories per pound. Starch is bad because it continually signals you to take another bite. Fat and protein signal your body to stop eating after a certain point, but carbohydrates, whether good or bad, don't. In nature, you had to eat prodigious amounts of them to get enough calories to stay alive, so a full stomach was the only shutoff signal you needed.

Even though the starch we eat today comes packed with calories, there's still no "turnoff" signal when you've eaten enough. Worse than that, it sparks a short-term surge of renewed hunger shortly after you eat. Starch is addictively appealing, packed with calories, has virtually no real nutritional value and makes you ravenous again thirty minutes after you eat.

Starch is so bad for you because it's basically sugar, and sugar plays a key role in how your body "reads" its own food supply. Briefly, the accumulation of sugar tells your body how much you just ate. That sounds odd, but it's true, and here's why it's important. The chemicals you use to digest food are powerful and dangerous. They are designed to destroy and absorb the things you eat, like meat. That means they can destroy parts of you, too. Gastric acid, for instance, can burn right through your stomach wall, and too much insulin—a critical agent of digestion—can kill you in no time. So you need to secrete just the right amount of acid and insulin to digest the food you ate. No less, because you need to absorb all the energy you can, but certainly no more, because you don't want to start digesting yourself. And you need some reliable signal from the food you ate to regulate the flow of those digestive elements.

Sugar is that signal. In nature, sugar content was closely proportional to the available fat and protein in each meal, and the ratio was surprisingly steady across most plant and animal species. The rise in free sugar in the bloodstream after a meal was a remarkably accurate indicator of how many calories were just consumed. That's why it became the most important control signal for your digestion. Not the only one, but the most important one. The amount of free sugar in food is known as the glycemic index, and it's a critical marker of nutrition. It's not listed on packages, but diabetics who take their disease seriously know glycemic numbers cold.

Since there isn't much free sugar in nature, a small rise in sugar signals the end of a pretty big meal. And remember, the whole digestive cascade—insulin and all—keys off these changes in blood sugar.

But this carefully balanced response, developed over hundreds of millions of years by fish, birds and dinosaurs, goes haywire in a fast-food world. Think back to when we were hunter-gatherers. Before we invented agriculture, we ate over two hundred different plants, fruits and nuts, and as many as a hundred different game animals, snakes, worms and insects. There was precious little starch or sugar in any of them. Grains like wheat and root vegetables like potatoes, which are phenomenally high in starch, are the creations of agriculture, introduced only 10,000 years ago. That feels like a long time to us, but it's a nonevent in the evolution of our digestive tracts.

For a long time, we could barely harvest enough of the stuff to survive. But now we have a vast excess. And, in combination with sedentary living and saturated fat, it is killing us.

Here's something to think about at dinner tonight. There's more free sugar (the stuff that flows right into your bloodstream to trigger your digestive response) in mashed potatoes than in table sugar. And here's something else. There's as much free sugar in a single can of cola as in five pounds of venison. And what about this? There's more free sugar—to say nothing of saturated fat—in a supersize side of fries than in five pounds of elk. How does your body respond? With confusion. Because the signal you send with a 1,000-calorie meal of soda, fries and a burger is that you have just eaten 10,000 calories of "natural food." And your body goes nuts, rushing out insulin and other digestive chemicals in response.

That's the real problem with starch. You have called for ten times the amount of digestive power you actually need. Ten times the insulin, gastric acid and a few dozen other dangerous chemicals. And things start to happen. First you hyperabsorb every last calorie from the food you ate. Second, because you obviously just killed a huge animal, your body tries to store every excess scrap of energy as fat. Third, because you now have enough insulin to digest a large animal but have killed only a soda and some fries, your blood sugar plummets and you're hungry again. Very, very hungry, and so you eat, usually quite a lot. What your poor Darwinian body reads is that you've gone from gluttony to starvation and back to gluttony in a couple of hours—*and it has no possible explanation for this!* This ultra-rapid cycling between gluttony and starvation has no parallel in nature. We talk about the signals you send with exercise, or by being sedentary, but our modern diet is so far outside your original design parameters that you are not sending *any* coherent signal. The whole system breaks down in a welter of hyperabsorption and decay. It's like rock stars smashing their guitars onstage. Noise comes out, but no more music. Adult diabetes is one of the results of this breakdown. Obesity, arthritis, heart disease, cancer and stroke are some of the others.

So back to the simple message. *Do not go on a diet, but quit eating crap.* No matter what else you do, cut out the junk. Cut out the starch and the sugar, and replace them with fruits, vegetables and whole grains—primitive, unrefined grains like pumpernickel and seven-grain bread. Quit eating more than you want. Say no to supersize portions, whether it's fries at the fast-food place or popcorn at the movies. Seriously consider ordering an appetizer and a salad as your full meal. Even that is usually more calories than you need, but it's a start.

Fat for Fuel

Now that you know how the insulin surge from eating starch drives your body to absorb every last calorie and store it as fat, it's only appropriate to start thinking about fat. And fat is going to surprise you. It has three roles in your body, and spilling over your belt is the least of them. You think of fat as storage, as that lump around your middle that grows steadily, year after year. But in nature fat is supposed to be active, dynamic tissue. The only time it turns into that inert lump is when winter comes. Active fat is healthy, essential, wonderful stuff. It's the inert fat of winter that does us in.

First, let's look at *active* fat, which we absorb and burn up every day, fat that we might store for a few hours, or a couple of days, but that moves in and out of our bodies as easily as it does in migrating birds flying to Africa. It's the healthy, "unsaturated" fat you've been hearing about. This fat, which is supposed to be the majority of the fat you consume, is the basic fuel for your metabolism and a key building block for your body.

Your body depends on the steady energy that fat supplies night and day throughout your life, and that's how you start to lose weight with exercise. Think of the hundredfold surge in C-6 that comes with running a marathon, and then the flooding river of C-10 that comes after it—the wave of inflammation that rips out all the tired, damaged muscle. The ensuing wave of growth that sweeps through your body, rebuilding your muscles and carrying the signals to grow into every corner of your body. That's all fueled by fat.

The wave of repair and regeneration goes on for hours after exercise, and your body runs in high gear the whole time, burning extra fat to replenish the energy in your muscles, to rebuild the glucose stores and the tissue so you can hunt again tomorrow. You burn far more fat recovering from exercise than you ever will on the treadmill. It's the great hidden trick to weight loss—stepping out of the gym, but still running your metabolism hard for the rest of the day. And even after the regeneration is complete and the muscles are rebuilt and recharged, your metabolism keeps ticking over at a higher rate than it does for the sedentary guys—even while you're sleeping. Your muscles are meat, not metal. You can't park them in the garage overnight, you have to feed them twenty-four hours a day. Sedentary men gain weight eating 2,000 calories a day; serious athletes, in peak condition, can lose weight eating 4,000 calories a day. Olympic athletes and

Navy SEALS in basic training struggle to avoid losing weight eating 6,000 calories a day. You're not going to get there, but you can probably increase your resting metabolic demand by 50 percent with good, stiff, daily exercise. That is key. You can achieve up to a 50 percent increase in your basal metabolism through vigorous exercise. That's how you lose weight.

Fat for Growth

Not only do you burn unsaturated fat, but you build with it. Your cell walls, for instance, all 40 billion of them, are largely fat, as are all the connections between our brain cells, our sex hormones and many of our chemical messenger molecules. You couldn't live a moment without the scaffolding of healthy fat that supports each living cell in your body. Indeed, you can't make a new cell without fat, and you make new cells all the time—more than twenty billion a year— especially when you're getting younger.

Your body is a massive, ongoing construction project, and unsaturated fat is one of the key building materials.

Fat for Storage

The fat that dominates our diet today is saturated fat—the form of fat we use to store energy for hard times. In nature, it's great stuff—an incredibly light and compact way to store energy. That might seem a little counterintuitive looking down at your belly, but it's true. Fat stores about twice as much energy per pound as sugar does. Another surprise, again counterintuitive in a Dunkin' Donuts world, is

The Good Fat

The dominant fat found in nature is unsaturated fat. It moves in and out of our bodies easily, burns cleanly as fuel and builds strong, resilient cells and tissues. Unsaturated fat, a mainstay of the natural diet we no longer eat, is found in wild-game meat, most vegetable oils (especially olive and canola oils), nuts, fruits, vegetables and especially fatty fish like mackerel, salmon and sardines. In our primitive diet, 30 percent of our calories came from fat, but it was mostly good, healthy, unsaturated fat. Ironically, our modern diet also gets about 30 percent of its calories from fat, but it's mostly the bad, unhealthy, saturated fat.

We have less unsaturated fat in our diet for two reasons. The first is economic. Free-range animals have only about 10 percent body fat, and it's mostly unsaturated. Once you ship them to the feedlot, keep them from moving and fatten them up, their percentage of body fat goes up to 30, and most of that is saturated. Profits zoom (there's a lot more money in a fat cow than a skinny one), but so do your weight and cholesterol. So cut way, way down on your consumption of red meat. Limit yourself to lean cuts and smaller sizes . . . and don't eat too much of them, either.

The other problem with unsaturated fat is that it goes rancid faster than saturated fat. It's not storage fat; it's active fat, ready to use throughout your body, but harder to store and ship. So the food industry—rationally enough from their point of view—has taken it out of our diets as much as possible. Unsaturated fat has become a trickle in our diets, accounting for a tiny percent of what it did when we lived in nature.

the fact that, in nature, even this fat comes off you with comparative ease. In modern life, however, in the perpetual winter we have created through sloth and gluttony, your body uses every possible trick to lay down extra calories as saturated fat and to hold on to them like grim death.

Saturated fat has the longest shelf life, both in your body and in the Oreos on the supermarket shelf; it's warehouse fat. That's why the food industry loves it. Those people don't hate you, or want you to die young; they just love that saturated fat is chemically stable, has a long shelf life and carries flavor well. Too bad your body likes the shelf life, too.

And now for some more bad news. Saturated fat is not a passive player; it's an inflammatory messenger in its own right, an automatic signal that it's time to decay. Add it into the diet of lab animals, and they immediately start to produce C-6. Obese people are five times more likely to have inflammatory proteins in their blood than lean people, and the most sedentary people, even controlling for body weight, are four times more likely to have inflammatory proteins in their blood than the most fit. Inflammatory proteins, remember, are the ones that can kill you with heart attacks, strokes and cancer. Which is why rates of prostate, colon, breast and ovarian cancers in populations around the world are directly proportional to dietary levels of saturated fat.

It's because winter never lasted for decades before, and C-6 never lasted for decades before either. Blood markers of inflammation, such as C-reactive protein (not coincidentally, a marker of heart attack risk), rise progressively with obesity, which makes sense: being sedentary triggers C-6, which tells your body to start laying down fat. The fat in turn triggers more C-6, leading to more decay and more fat deposits, which triggers more C-6 . . . and so on. In response, white blood cells invade your fat tissue, creating a pool of decay, and then the white blood cells themselves secrete their own C-6, creating a vicious and deadly cycle of fat-inflammation-fat-inflammation. Even worse, your fat tissue secretes C-6 faster the fatter you get.

C-6 also makes it harder for your body to listen to the changes you do make in your diet. Researchers have found that mice, and patients, with high levels of systemic inflammation, those headed fastest toward their heart attacks, are the most resistant to cholesterol reductions with diet. Up to 40 percent of the cells in fat tissue in an obese person are not fat cells at all, but rather inflammatory cells—the same white blood cells we talked about in the walls of your arteries. And they release a steady trickle of C-6 day and night, but never enough to trigger C-10. You might hear the C-6 if you listen carefully when you open the refrigerator door in the middle of the night: *hiss-bump, hiss-bump.*

Is all this sounding familiar? It should, from reading about heart attacks in Chapter Five. Disturbingly familiar. The same white blood cells that invade your arterial walls to form plaque invade your fat tissue to cause the inflammation of chronic obesity. Even the minimum maintenance repair cycles begin to break down. Without enough unsaturated fat to build with, an obese person's body substitutes saturated fat. It builds the stuff right into your cell walls. But it's a slightly different shape than unsaturated fat and it doesn't quite fit. Imagine building a wall where some of the bricks are just a little off: that would be your cell walls. And so they don't work quite right. The other problem is that the saturated fat is still inflammatory, triggering local inflammation, which produces tiny drops of C-6 that collect throughout the cell walls of your most important tissues. Let me say it again: *Heart disease, stroke, cancer and even Alzheimer's disease are all strongly linked to the inflammation caused by the saturated fat in our diet.*

Saturated fat (and cholesterol) are found in full-fat dairy (butter, cheese, milk and cream), but skim milk, nonfat yogurt and nonfat cheese are pretty good for you. Eggs are probably fine in moderation, though no one knows for sure, and meat is generally bad. Very lean cuts of beef and pork are okay but hard to come by, and bacon and sausage, which I love, are terrible. You also have to steer clear of trans fat, a hidden, artificial fat the food industry came up with. Functionally, it's just the same as saturated fat, but it won't show up on most food labels for another couple of years. It's in every fried food, every doughnut, every cookie, pie, pastry and almost every cracker you can buy in America. Pick up a bag of potato chips and add up all the fats listed on the label. Then look at the total fat number. They won't match. The "missing" fat is the trans fat. And it's very, very bad for you.

That's enough on the dark side for this short primer on nutrition, but I hope the core message is clear. Stop eating crap. Eat less. And exercise *hard* six days a week.

What *Can* You Eat?

Get ready for a quick canter through a list of the good guys. Go as heavy as you can on fruits, vegetables and *whole* grains. That's important for two reasons: fiber and micronutrients. Fiber is simple. It's roughage—indigestible roughage. It slows down the absorption of fat and keeps your colon working, clean and free of cancer. It's also the bulk you need to fill you up so you feel like you had a square meal. We had a ton of it in our original diets but have almost none now. Fiber content is listed on packages, so read those labels. High-fiber cereals and breads have about three grams per serving. Since your goal should be about forty grams a day, you can see how far we have to go.

Micronutrients, mainly trace minerals and vitamins, are also important . . . and just a little odd. There are hundreds of them, and no one knows for sure how much of each we need. We know they are critical to thousands of chemical reactions in our bodies and in short supply in our modern diets. We know they include chemicals that are essential to our immune systems, muscle and brain function, heart health, bone health and blood formation, as well as the antioxidants that protect us against cancer. We know they abound in fruit and vegetables, and that you can't get them from supplements. In addition, we know that individual needs differ. Your body needs a slightly different mix of micronutrients than Chris's body or your neighbor's body. But there is no way to figure out which ones you need, or in what concentrations (though you can spend thousands of dollars getting your hair, fingernails, urine and blood analyzed by people who will tell you differently). So take that multivitamin, but don't fool yourself into thinking that a breakfast of vitamin pills substitutes in any way for a healthy diet. Instead, eat a wide variety of good stuff, and your body will pick and choose what it needs with unerring accuracy.

The latest official recommendation is to eat nine servings a day of fruits and vegetables. Yes, it's a huge amount of leafy stuff, but work at it. Your colon may even start acting normally again! It makes very little difference which ones you eat, but try to eat at least four different colors of fruits and vegetables each day (shades of green count). And don't listen to people who malign fruit on account of its sugar content. That's nonsense. Fruit is loaded with nutrients, and in the context of the sugar load of our modern diets, worrying about the downside of fruit is silly.

Whole grains and legumes (beans) are the other major healthy food category. Before grains are processed, they contain a broad range of nutrients and not much free sugar. (Refining flour breaks down the cell walls of the grains and releases the sugar, which is why it makes food taste so good. But it also strips out most of the micronutrients and fiber.) Most "whole wheat" and multigrain bread in the supermarket doesn't count as truly whole-grain, which you'll understand if you read the labels. The first ingredient in the supermarket "health" breads is unbleached but *refined* flour. (Bleaching it makes it into white bread, but it's the refining part that turns it into starch.) The only good stuff is the heavy bread that comes from the health food store—seven-grain, twelve-grain, pumpernickel and so forth. Whole grains (whole wheat, whole rye, etc.) have to be the *first* thing on the ingredients list, not the last, or someone is misleading you. Whole-grain breads have richer flavors than refined-flour breads, so it doesn't take long to get used to them and come to like them. (Refined flour does not taste any better; it's just that you're used to the sugar, and sugar is an acquired taste.) Luckily, as you get older, your taste buds don't like sugar as much and you can appreciate other flavors. You *can* get used to coffee with no sugar (or at least coffee with fewer than ten sugars); it takes only a month or so. Breakfast cereals are an easy place to win with this. Cheerios have whole wheat as the first ingredient, followed by things you don't need, but are still respectable. Shredded wheat has only one ingredient: whole wheat! Add some skim milk and a banana, or frozen blueberries, and you're a third of the way toward a healthy day.

Protein will not be a problem if you come even vaguely near a healthy diet . . . especially if you force yourself to like skim milk and other nonfat dairy. (Again, give it a month.) Eat lots of fish, the oilier the better. Eat white meat chicken, too: not as great as fish, but much better than red meat. Obviously, you're going to eat some red meat—this is America, after all, and it does taste wonderful—but take it easy. Eat much, much less, and get it as lean as you can, especially for burgers. In fact, start thinking of meat as a flavoring rather than a staple; a little bit goes a long way.

Salt is also pretty easy to discuss: we eat too much of it. We're supposed to get two grams a day, but most of us get eight to ten without even lifting a salt shaker. Since food manufacturers add salt and sugar to everything they make, just stay as close to fresh foods as you can and never add salt again.

One more tip: Make a copy of the Harvard food pyramid on page 200 and put it on the refrigerator door. Food purveyors like to say there's no such thing as bad food, there's just sometimes too much. Well, that's not quite right. Some things are so much worse for you that it makes sense to see them as just plain bad. Look at the pyramid. The good ones are near the bottom.

Remember, if you buy it, you will eventually eat it. Good nutrition happens in the supermarket, not in the kitchen. Eat a good meal before you shop, make a list of all the healthy stuff you want to buy and take a quick look at the food pyramid as you head out the door. Guess what? You will be thinner next year.

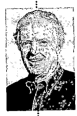

CHAPTER SIXTEEN

"The Drink"

n Ireland, the people have a special relationship with whiskey and other strong waters. They call it "The Drink," with capital letters in their voices. As one might say: "Then it was The Drink, I suppose, that took him away, the dear man." As if to explain that the departed had been in the grip of forces larger than himself and was not entirely to blame. Being a quarter Irish myself, I have a wary respect for The Drink. And a deep and abiding affection for it, too. As for a wonderfully amusing old uncle—or perhaps a charming niece—who once in a great, great while . . . murders someone. Once a month, say, but nothing you can't forgive in someone who is so much fun the rest of the time.

The Drink is such a joker in the deck of our lives that it is hard to know what, if anything, to say about it. Harry thinks it's so scary that we shouldn't talk about it at all, because, if you're going to talk about it, you have to mention the good side and that can be dangerously misleading for some guys. He worries that they'll just hear what they want to hear and tumble into addiction. Harry says, if alcohol were a medicine and had the side effects that it does—i.e., maybe 20 percent of users become *abusers* at some point in their lives—it would never get FDA approval. My reaction is respectful, as always of Harry's views, but a little different.

First, wine and liquor have FDA approval and have had it for about ten thousand years. They tried to change that during Prohibition, and it didn't work so well. It's here; it's already in most of our lives; and it's not going away. So it makes sense to talk about it. Second, there is the troubling but stubborn fact that, for some of us, wine and liquor are among the great joys of life. Third, there are some remarkable population studies that indicate that drinking *in moderation* (you'll want to remember that part) is terrific for you. So, it is a tricky story, with the good news and bad news we've become so familiar with.

On the Bright Side

The good news is astonishing. I've been drinking for a while, but I was stunned, on New Year's Eve 2002, to read in *The New York Times,* and later in *Scientific American,* that steady drinking in moderation (which means two drinks or less a day for men; one for women) is not just fun . . . it is powerful medicine. (Before you get too excited, a "drink" is one and a half ounces of booze, or five ounces of wine.) Booze, used regularly and in moderation, is terrific for just about everything that ails you. Not, let me quickly say, if you become an alcoholic. Then it kills you. And lots and lots of perfectly nice men do become low-level (and high-level) alcoholics in their sixties and seventies; that's what scares Harry. But, in moderation, it is good for you. There are so many of these studies, and the results are so clear, that it is hard to argue with them, unless you want to step onto some kind of religious or moral ground. Here's some of what I read that day in the *Times*:

"Alcohol has become the sharpest double-edged sword in medicine. Thirty years of research has convinced many experts of the health benefits of moderate drinking for some people. A drink or two a day of wine, beer or liquor is, experts say, often the single best nonprescription way to prevent heart attacks—better than a low-fat diet or weight loss, better even than vigorous exercise. Moderate drinking can help prevent strokes, amputated limbs and dementia." (Amputated limbs? Yup, amputated limbs. Worth thinking about, for you clumsy do-it-your-selfers.)

The reporter, Abigail Zuger, went on: " 'The science supporting the protective role of alcohol is indisputable; no one questions it anymore,' said Dr. Curtis Ellison, a professor of medicine and public health at the Boston University School of Medicine. 'There have been hundreds of studies, all consistent.' "

"In a study of more than 80,000 American women, those who drank moderately had only half the heart attack risk of those who did not drink at all, even if they were slim, did not smoke and exercised daily."

"In thousands of middle-aged Danish men with high cholesterol, moderate drinkers had 50% less risk of developing heart disease from blocked arteries than abstainers."

"Among more than 100,000 California adults, moderate drinking after age 40 was associated with reduced death rates during every subsequent decade of life—in some people by as much as 30 percent."

Consider what Walter C. Willett, chairman of the Department of Nutrition at the Harvard School of Public Health, says in his *Eat, Drink, and Be Healthy*: "For men, study after study has shown that men who have one or two alcoholic drinks a day are 30 to 40 percent less likely to have heart attacks than men who don't drink alcohol at all. That's about the same as seen for the powerful cholesterol-lowering drugs known as statins. . . . Having more than two drinks a day further increases the heart and stroke protection but also increases the chances the dark side of alcohol will emerge." The January 2002 issue of *Scientific American* made basically the same points, citing different studies.

The *Times* piece pointed out that the studies at last explained the endlessly pleasing "French paradox," which arises from the fact that the French eat more cheese, butter and other fats than you can shake a stick at, and still "their hearts are relatively free of fatty blockage." This also explains the Italian or Mediterranean paradox, to say nothing of the Chris Crowley paradox. It is good to have these things cleared up. Harry takes a wary, if not actually hostile view of the pleasing French and other paradoxes. He suspects bad science in there somewhere. I, on the other hand, suspect his Puritan roots.

It doesn't matter what you drink. There is still some lingering thought that red wine is a damn fine antidote to cancer, but in general it doesn't matter. As long as you're steady about it. Drink a little every day, they all say. No bunching up . . . no bingeing. Every day. I imagine your wife sticking her head into your study: "Honey, have you had your martini yet?" Or, *"Drink your wine, damn you! Do you want to die?"*

So, there you are . . . what all of us should have known all along. Wine and beer and booze are marvelous for us. At last, the scientific community is talking some sense.

The Dark Side

Okay, so *The New York Times, Scientific American* and Dr. Willett do make oblique reference to teeny problems associated with *too much* alcohol. In fact, they say the risk of too much alcohol takes quite a lot of the fun out of the good news. And the notion of what is too much cuts in pretty early.

From that same *Times* piece: "Heavy drinking raises the risk of high blood pressure, heart failure and half a dozen forms of cancer; it may cause diabetes, pancreatic failure, liver failure and severe dementia. Heavy drinkers have mortality rates far higher than moderate drinkers, statistics which do not even include the effects of car accidents and alcohol-fueled violence that destroy not only the drinker but others as well."

Then they go on to make the dreary point that "The net health effects of alcohol are heavily influenced by its dangers. The World Health Organization estimates that over all, alcohol causes as much illness and death as measles and malaria, and more years of life lost to death and disability than tobacco or illegal drugs." Not so great.

In other words, it appears that there are serious advantages and serious risks. And, in fairness, you should know that the risks may get more grave as you get older. As you have doubtless noticed, it takes less booze to make you stupid now. And you may be better placed to become an alcoholic in retirement, because there is less structure in your life and, for some, more stress. So you get a new shot, in your sixties, at becoming a drunk. A fairly good shot, in Harry's experience. And it doesn't just happen to dopes and losers, he says. Successful, solid guys with stable families and all that suddenly take a funny turn. Happens a lot. So do not assume you can handle The Drink just because you've been doing so for the last forty years or because you're a great guy. It may not be true. Watch it.

I hate to do this, but I have to expand a bit on the sad notion that less booze makes you more stupid as you get older. We all have deeply ingrained ideas in our heads of "normal" eating and "normal" drinking. In the Next Third, normal eating will make you fat; normal drinking will make you drunk. It's as simple as that, and as bad. We really, really have to change the rules in our heads on both fronts or we'll get into trouble. Sorry. Two drinks a day is a *real* maximum for most men in the Next Third. Hard to believe, but true.

You may be pleased to know that if you *do* become a drunk in your sixties, you probably won't wind up on the streets. Harry's my source on this, too, and he says the likelihood is that the late-blooming drunk will be a "high-functioning alcoholic." Congratulations. That means you will be moseying down life's highway looking like an idiot, talking nonsense and not doing much . . . one of those country club drunks with plaid pants and a purple nose. Or the retired guy sitting in the dark, staring at the TV in the middle of the afternoon, utterly whacked. Not a good use of the Next Third of your life.

I hate to mention it, but addiction or alcoholism is not the only downside to drinking. Harry recently sent me a story on a study of heavy but functioning nonalcoholic drinkers. Men who drank a little more than three glasses of wine a night were shown in MRI tests to have measurable brain damage. "Our heavy drinkers sample was significantly impaired in measures of working memory, processing speed, attention, executive function, and balance," according to researcher Dieter Meyerhoff in the May 2004 *Journal of Alcoholism.* "Heavy drinking damages your brain ever so slightly, reducing your cognitive functioning in ways that may not be readily noticeable. To be safe, don't overdo it." In other words, while a little booze is good, more than a little is bad. And the sweet spot is pretty small.

My trainer made a terrifying point about drinking the other day. I was feeling puny, I told him, because I'd had most of a bottle of wine the night before. I couldn't lift as much or do as many reps as usual. "That figures," he said. "Drinking too much ages you." *What?* Here I am, working like a crazy man to be younger, and my beloved Drink is making me old? Yep, it's true.

Okay, here is my serious, bottom-line advice, which is similar to what the experts say. If you don't drink, don't start. Too risky. That's mainstream advice. If you do drink, don't stop—*if you're able to do it in moderation.* Which is not so easy. If you *are* able to drink in moderation, you're golden. But remember, the cutoff point is two drinks a night, and that's not many. As few as three-plus glasses of wine a night, over time, is bad.

Here is the golden mean to which I aspire, sometimes with success, sometimes not: Have a glass or two of wine a night as a magical garnish with your meal. A gentle push into a pleasant evening. Perhaps one night a week, feel free to have three. And quit. If you notice the "gentle push" getting a teeny bit urgent—like an old pet that is suddenly starting to growl and act funny—stop. 'Cause that sucker can bite you in a heartbeat, and the wound can fester for the rest of your life. At our age, things can get a lot worse a lot faster than we imagine.

But at our age, we also need as much joy as we can get our mitts on. For me, that most assuredly includes a glass or two of wine most nights, until death. Occasionally the exquisite, the life-enhancing martini. Possibly two.

PART TWO

Take Charge of Your Life

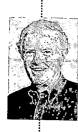

CHAPTER SEVENTEEN

"Teddy Doesn't Care!"

W hen I was sent off to first grade in the fall of 1940— to the very same school Harry was sent to a hundred years later—my father and my Uncle Ben (two men of tremendous energy and charm) had me pumped. They cared like crazy, and they passed it on. I was urged to grab a seat in the first row on the first day, which I did. I was told to listen hard and to get my hand up fast, and I did that, too. I duked it out with Deedee Bethell for the monthly spelling prize, which went mostly to her but sometimes to me. That delighted Pa and Uncle Ben.

One kid named Teddy took a different line. He sat in the back and was not much interested in what was going on. When pressed by the teacher one day, he astonished me by saying, with perfect serenity, "I don't care." That was it. The teacher let it go. I went home that afternoon, absolutely flabbergasted. I told Pa and Uncle Ben and the others, "Teddy doesn't care!" Again and again, that day and later, "Teddy does *not* care!" I couldn't get over it. The phrase became a joke in my family. My beloved sister Petie still says it sometimes, when I press her to do this or that and she doesn't want to. "Teddy doesn't care," she says and ruefully shakes her head. Won't budge after that. It still stumps me.

At this stage, you may think that I must have been a *nightmare* as a child. And as an old man. True. But think about this: *Caring* . . . being interested enough to get up every day and give it a shot . . . to do new stuff, do old stuff . . . to keep on going when you wouldn't mind sitting down for a while . . . that is a gift of God. Or Darwin. Or The Shore Country Day School. It is *the* great theme of this entire book, and a true blessing. At some juncture, some dark and stormy night when you can't sleep, some dreary Monday morning when you've lost interest in yourself and others, there is an almost irresistible temptation to say, "Who gives a shit?" And really, who does? Who cares if you get up and do your exercises today? Or eat a vast tub of popcorn at the movies? Or work on that project you've been so excited about? Really, who actually gives a shit?

I respectfully submit that the answer better be "I do." Or you're cooked. That is the message of the last few chapters of the book in particular, which is why it rises to the level of being Harry's Sixth Rule. Harry's Sixth Rule reads, in its entirety: *Care.*

Care is a triple-barreled message, a Gatling gun of advice. First, we urge you to care enough about exercise and nutrition so that you have a decent body and a good attitude going into the Next Third. Lord knows, that's important. But mostly the book veers off into new territory at this point and we mean something a little different. Up until now, it has almost all been about your body and being *physically* younger next year. Critical stuff, obviously, and the foundation for the rest of your life. But that's only part of it, and not necessarily the most important part. With exercise, you have given yourself a great set of wheels. But that doesn't amount to much unless you go out on the road. The rest of the book is about life on the road. Once you've taken charge of your body, you have to think about taking charge of your life.

We believe that getting out on the road in the Next Third means reconnecting and recommitting to other people. As a matter of fact, that's Harry's Seventh Rule: *Connect and commit*. It means rededicating yourself to family, friends, companions. Get involved in groups and do communal things, whether work or play. There is a strong temptation to do less on this front as we age, but that is a huge mistake. Because, it turns out, we were literally built to be involved with and to care for one another, and that does not change one bit as we age. That's what being a mammal is all about. That's Harry's next chapter, and it is powerful stuff. If we don't exercise our social skills— if we let ourselves become cut off and increasingly solitary as we age—we will become ill and die. Hundreds of fascinating studies demonstrate the point. So "caring" means caring about other people and being involved with them . . . acting like the pack animals we are, right to the end.

The next suggestion goes beyond that. It is a recommendation that we get involved in a kind of caring that satisfies what may be a core element of our rational brain as well as our essential human character. We believe that we were built to aspire to things beyond the interests of ourselves or our immediate pack . . . to "care" in that exalted sense. There is at least a possibility that this "higher caring" is what being a human and having a reasoning mind is all about.

Harry and I don't want to say too much about higher caring, which can range from working in a soup kitchen to building cathedrals, because it is so very personal. For many people, choosing how they want to work for the greater good is influenced by their notions of spirituality, a topic we simply can't deal with seriously within the compass of this book. But we can say that finding the selflessness within you—getting that one right for you—may trump everything else. Caring at every level is one of the most important things you can do in the Next Third of your life.

Keep a Log or Lose Your Command

Back to earth and some mundane advice about the *mechanics* of caring. One of the great keys to caring about your own life is to *watch it*. And to keep track as if it mattered a lot. Which it does. If you're going to have a good life, a full life, a life that you and others care about, it must be *the examined life*. And that means writing stuff down. It sounds banal, but it works. It's so easy to look out at the rain and give it the Full Teddy—"I don't care"—and go back to sleep. If you know you're going to have to admit it, in writing, you're more likely to get up and go.

So keep a simple log in which you write down, every stinking day, these three things: 1) what I ate, 2) what I did for exercise (or didn't), and 3) what I did with my life—sexually, socially, morally . . . whatever lights your fire. It is a tremendous help to know, as you decide from minute to minute what to do, that "All Will Be Written" and "All Will Be Known." It is a talismanic business, a sign that *someone cares*. Even if it's just you.

Keeping the log—and keeping it accurately—has been the sacred duty of captains and commanders from the earliest times. Those who tampered with or kept a false log faced grave penalties, certainly including loss of command. That's a good phrase, actually. If you do not keep an accurate log, you will lose command. Of yourself.

I first learned this log stunt from my passionate one-on-one diet adviser, Stephen Gullo. He had a sensible regimen and a hundred clever tricks. But his first trick was that he cared. His real trick was that he taught me to care. And his most important device was the keeping of a log.

Every day I had to fill in a sheet, listing every damn thing I ate or drank, and then fax it to him. Once a week, I had to go sit in his office while he lectured and cheered me on. After he and I were done, I kept up my log and became my own cheering section. I already knew what not to eat; everyone does. The big thing was teaching myself to care. The price of fitness is eternal vigilance, and the greatest spur to diligence is the daily log. Works equally well with your efforts to connect and commit. Write stuff down and you become a serious man, in the sense of someone who cares. A daily log is a crutch to lean on when you're weak. A shield to ward off boredom when you're tired. A sword to symbolize your resolve when you falter. It is a practical tool and a magical device that stands between you and the relentless thought "You know what? I just don't care." A couple of times I lost my log and, *without fail,* went straight to hell. In my experience, there is a perfect correlation between dropping the log and going to hell. So now I carry it everywhere. And I keep it religiously.

But whether you try it or not, remember: The great trick in life is to care. On the surface and at the deep heart's core. Teddy died young, by the way. Teddy didn't care.

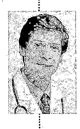

CHAPTER EIGHTEEN

The Limbic Brain and the Biology of Emotion

U p to this point, the book has been about our bodies and
how to grow physically younger for years to come.
Now we want to talk about the emotional and mental
sides of our lives, because many of the choices we make
there have just as much biological impact as the choices
we make for our physical bodies. Staying emotionally connected, in particular, turns out to be a biological imperative,
a critical part of the good life—and a real challenge as we
age in our society.

In general, men don't do such a great job of staying connected to people, or of living fully as they get older. Men
think they can separate reason and emotion, mind and heart,
thinking and feeling. Having performed that remarkable
trick, they think they can put the emotional side on the back
burner, or ignore it completely, and they tend to believe they
will be better men as a result. This is a mistaken notion. It

is not a good idea, and it is not possible. It is unhealthy and delusional; it goes directly against the grain of how we were made.

We evolved as social pack animals, like wolves and dolphins. It's not a choice; our survival depends on being part of a group. No one has ever gone into the Amazon jungle and found an isolated person; it's always a tribe. There is no such thing as a solitary human in nature, because isolation is fatal. We were designed to be emotional creatures, which is to say that we are mammals.

"So what?" you ask. "Why is being a mammal so special?" After all, a hundred million years ago we were furry, insignificant little rodents, trying not to get stepped on by dinosaurs, barely holding on to our evolutionary niche. We are special, and we triumphed, because we invented a second brain.

Remember the primitive, reptilian brain? The extraordinary, runs-your-body-perfectly, does-exactly-what-you-tell-it-to brain? Well, mammals built a whole new brain that sits right on top of the reptilian one. You can think of it as the emotional brain, but its real name is the limbic brain. Roll that word around on your tongue: *limbic*. You're going to find it coming up over and over again in your conversations after you finish this book. Chris now uses the word incessantly and enjoys it immensely. It's an actual, physical chunk of brain that runs our emotions, and in many ways it's the most important brain you have. You can scoop this brain up and hold it in your hand. You can see it work with functional MRI scanning. You can trace its development back a hundred million years. Complex emotions, from the limbic brain, are the reason mammals succeeded—the reason we survived when the dinosaurs did not. We are social and emotional creatures from start to finish.

Fear and Anger, Love and Play

Your physical, reptilian brain has the control centers for fear and aggression, our deepest and most primitive emotions. Killing prey, territorial defense, fight or flight, sexual predation and ruthless self-interest are the legacy of our earliest ancestors. Reptiles developed our primal negative emotions. Surges of adrenaline, morphine, serotonin and scores of other chemicals flood the crocodile's brain when the prey dives into the river. We have that brain and those chemicals today. They are our automatic, chemical responses to the environment, to threat or prey, and they work!

The brilliance, the absolute triumph of mammals, is that we took the same chemistry, the same neurological pathways, the same wiring, and turned it around to create positive emotions. Reptiles run purely on negative reinforcement. Mammals invented love, joy, pleasure and play, all of which are enshrined in our DNA, in the chemical and neurological pathways in our limbic brains.

But the reptiles were doing pretty well with anger, fear and aggression. Why go further? What's the biological point of love or friendship, of being happy, sad, optimistic or enthusiastic? Why invest extra energy in building a whole new level of brain structures? The answer is, to work together.

Nature hardwired our reptilian ancestors for their own *individual* survival. Apart from a drive to have sex, reptiles have no parental instinct. Most of them cheerfully eat their young, which is why they're programmed to lay eggs and get out of town before they hatch. Remember, reptilian instincts are still a deeply powerful part of us. Our primitive brain still runs our most basic functions, giving us a fierce, primal drive for our personal survival. What it doesn't give us is a concern for the survival of our children or the ability to sense the emotions of others.

Our limbic brain gives us two critical advantages over the reptiles. It lets us love our young and work in groups. Its first and most powerful creation is the emotional cascade triggered by the sight and sounds of our own offspring. The overwhelming biology of parental love swamps our more basic, selfish instincts—don't eat the baby! As time went by, the limbic tool kit allowed us to build a complex neurological array of positive reinforcement for the sharing of food, warmth, shelter, information and parenting.

Parenting and Living in Packs

Mammals succeeded because we learned how to invest much more in our young than lizards do. "Don't get between a mother bear and her cubs" is wisdom known to all of us. But the words "Don't get between a turtle and her eggs" have never appeared in print before.

Live young take much more energy before birth than eggs do, and actually sticking around to raise the young takes even more investment in each offspring. "Prey mammals," like mice, have a relatively modest commitment to their young. They have large, frequent litters and expect to lose quite a few from each. Genetically, they are protected by their numbers more than by their parents. Predator mammals, like bears and humans, on the other hand, have few offspring, take a long time to raise them to independence and safety, and are profoundly connected to them. The loss of a predator child is a major genetic blow to the parent, and the limbic brain drives a much greater emotional attachment as a result.

Here's a critical point. Your limbic brain is physically in control of your primitive brain and deeply wired into it, but it's only in *partial* control. It has a series of small control centers that sit on top of and around the physical brain. Each center is primarily responsible for different moods, but they are cross-wired so they talk to one another all the time. In a very real sense, your emotions and moods control your body's basic, physical chemistry.

Think of the physical reaction you have to anxiety. That's the limbic brain kicking your reptilian adrenaline into action, like a rider on a big, powerful horse with a mean streak. If the rider is good, he has a lot of control, but the horse will always be a bigger, stronger animal. If the rider isn't so good, or if the horse spooks, he can get thrown and the horse will take off without him. The same holds true for your primal instincts. If you work at it, your limbic brain can become a good, even great rider, but the horse will always outweigh you by a thousand pounds; you will never be as firmly in control as you would like to think. In practical terms, that means you will pay a steep physical price if you don't get the emotional structure of your life into fairly good shape.

Luckily for us, although the limbic brain responds to both positive and negative reinforcement, it responds best to the chemistry of pleasure. We feel good about our offspring and about being part of a working group. Back in nature, packs let us forage with a collective eye out for predators, hunt more effectively and share child-raising. Packs also let us sleep: a surprisingly important activity, which we spend a third of our lives at. Mammals can sleep at night and doze during the day because their limbic systems synchronize throughout the pack. At least one animal is always in light sleep and will wake the others if there is a threat. Reptiles can't synchronize their rhythms and therefore can't rely on a pack to let them sleep. They can never relax . . . never rely on the group to watch their back when their eyes are closed.

Sleep is still largely mysterious, but one of its major functions is to give our metabolisms downtime for routine maintenance, which is especially important because we are warm-blooded. Being warm-blooded lets us run at full speed whenever we want. We can hunt at night, or in the predawn chill, because we keep our muscles at 98.6 degrees, ready to go, all the time, but running at high speed all the time takes its toll. NASCAR drivers wear out a $75,000 engine with each race, and then it's back to the shop for a new one. We are not far off. When we're on high alert and stressed, we secrete a steady river of adrenaline and cortisol: our stress hormones. They keep us in high gear for the demands of kill-or-be-killed but, like the race car, at a cost. Our bodies need a constant repair effort, and it can only happen when we're not racing. In effect, adrenaline and cortisol prevent us from diverting energy to repair when we might need it to survive.

Some Practical Advice on Sleep

As you get older, you need about an hour less sleep a night, but that sleep is more important. The biological catch-22 is that you don't sleep as well as the years go on, which means you have to work harder at it. My advice is embarrassingly simple, but here it is: Go to bed an hour earlier than you usually do, in a room that's truly dark. Try it for a month and see how much your quality of life changes. The best way to ensure that you wake up halfway through the night and get poor-quality sleep is to drink alcohol in the evening, with caffeine after lunch a close second, so watch what you're drinking. Finally, if you don't get a good night's sleep, try to sneak in a nap after lunch.

When the environment is not threatening, when it's time to relax, another set of chemicals are released, like serotonin and relatives of morphine and Valium. These are the signals that it's safe to wind down and go into the shop to replace the engine, rebuild the transmission and get ready for tomorrow's race. This balance between high alert and repair mode fluctuates throughout the day, but the major repair period is when we sleep.

The downside of being warm-blooded is that we have to maintain a constant body temperature, which is not a trivial issue when the weather turns nasty. Snuggling is about as cheap (and beneficial) a way of heating yourself as possible. Mammals, it turns out, are actually drawn to one another— to physical, social contact. Touch produces serotonin, which feels good. We want more of it, and we seek out contact. The snuggling, the warm safety of the pack, releases more serotonin in our brains, and the serotonin blocks the release of adrenaline and cortisol. It's the physical signal that the hunt is over, that it's time to wind down. Time to let our body repair itself after a day of hunting, gathering and not being eaten. In the bad old days of evolution, being eaten or starving to death were not abstractions—they were daily realities. Striking the right balance between fear, high-alert mode and calm, relaxed, repair-and-feeding mode was critical. Emotions let us do this collectively rather than individually, which puts us a half-step ahead of the competition.

But the reptilian brain was always there, lurking below the surface of group living. *You*—the individual—still have to survive in order to reproduce. So the limbic brain and the reptilian brain learned to work together, balancing the individual with the pack. Balancing the primal emotions of fear and aggression with the new emotions of love, joy, pleasure and play. Being part of a pack takes constant positive reinforcement; if we don't experience it, if we isolate ourselves, the negative chemistry of our reptilian brain takes over. That's why play turns out to be such a surprisingly important mammalian achievement. It's a strong signal that we are part of a healthy group. Our limbic brain leads us to crave companionship for its own sake. To want to belong to and matter to those around us. To love, and to be loved in return.

Nature wastes nothing, and it never stops working, so let's give the limbic brain a hundred million years to grow up, and look what happens.

The Storyteller

Long, long ago, a wandering storyteller, powerfully built but dressed in ragged garments, joins your tribe in the small, close circle around the low, flickering fire. The night is clear and cool, and the stars are brilliant pinpricks of light in the darkness overhead. Beyond the light cast by the fire, the world is lost in shadow. Men and women sit together, their children leaning back against their knees, as the storyteller launches into his tale. Starting with a tone so low that you have to bend forward to hear him, he builds his tale of one man's love for a woman—a tale of betrayal, war and loneliness. As he speaks, he looks slowly and deliberately around the circle. His eyes meet yours across the fire, and you feel the physical shock of the connection. His eyes are deep-set, and as you look deeper into them his soft words become real and the story becomes yours. You fall in love with the heroine. You feel the hero's anguish and anger as she's stolen away. You join your brothers in vengeful preparation for war, and you lose yourself in the direct, primal connection with Ulysses as he sits across the fire and tells of the fall of Troy and of his long odyssey to return home.

So what happened around that fire? Why can we connect so deeply with others? Why can the person across the fire—or the table—affect your mood so powerfully, stir you to passion, anger, laughter or tears? You've had this experience. You know that friends, family, storytellers, musicians, actors—and audiences—all have this effect on your own moods and emotions. How does this work?

The explanation is, in the end, simple and physical. Because of the limbic way we're made, we are not emotional islands. Simply put, *we complete each other.* In both good and bad ways, to be sure, but we do complete each other, and therefore we cannot make it alone. This is such a magical part of being alive that it seems almost sacrilegious to look behind the curtain. But the biology turns out to be just as magical as the experience, fairly simple, and critical to the rest of your life.

Your limbic brain reads the real world and makes emotions out of it. We read hundreds of subtle signals in each encounter: body language, tone of voice, the flickers of facial expression that give nuance to each sentence, the glances that speak their own volumes. Neurologically, we are profoundly visual creatures. The visual processing centers in our brains are enormous—far out of proportion to our eyesight, which is about average as animals go. So why build all that extra brainpower around fairly puny signals? And what are you looking at, anyway?

It turns out that you don't devote much of your brain to looking at trees, or rocks, or even prey. You look at people. Specifically, you look at faces with a hungry intensity. Standard visual information about where the doorknob is, or how fast the tennis ball is moving, goes to a few, relatively small areas of your brain. When you look at another person, however, and specifically when you look at a person's face, functional MRI scanning shows massive sections of brain waking up to process the information. It's like someone throwing the switch for a night game at Yankee Stadium; a huge, brightly lit image shows up on the scan, totally separate from the area that processed the image of a rock, and it's all devoted to absorbing and interpreting every nuance of facial expression.

Sadly, autistic children (and, to a lesser degree, severely abused or neglected children and severely depressed patients) don't do this. The faces of those who love them register in the standard vision areas—in the most severe cases with no more limbic content than a street sign. Yankee Stadium remains dark and empty.

We are primarily visual creatures, but further floods of information come from sounds, from touch, smell, temperature, from all our myriad sensors, internal and external; the limbic brain is constantly supplied with an astonishingly rich stream of information about every aspect of what's happening inside and outside our bodies. There are millions of signals to the limbic brain, every second, and each one gets a tiny chemical tag, a minute emotion, as it moves through the brain. Scientists have yet to find *any* brain signal that does not get a specific emotional tag from your limbic systems.

How can your brain make sense of this staggering, impossible ocean of information? The solution is brilliantly simple. Your brain makes maps. And not just a few maps, but maps of everything—thousands of them every second. Physical, social and intellectual maps streaming in, emotional maps streaming out. To a large extent, you navigate your world and your life from emotional maps.

Sensory maps come up from the physical brain below: one map for temperature around the body, another map of light touch around the body (the feeling of a gentle breeze on your skin, or a light caress), another of visual information, a listening map, a map of salt concentration in your blood, of muscle position and tension, of bowel function, of bladder fullness, of saliva secretion, of scent—thousands more maps of individual, discrete physical patterns.

In addition, thousands of *social* maps come down from the thinking, social brain above—the brain that makes you human. Where do you stand in the pack, who owes you food or favors, whom can you trust, whom can you not, who likes you, whom do you like, what is every member of the group feeling, thinking and doing each second . . . hundreds of social calculations going on all the time.

And each map, each of the thousands of physical and social maps you create each second, also gets an emotional tag: a chemical feeling about your world. Each map contributes a slight chemical nuance to the limbic chemistry, a dash of serotonin, morphine or adrenaline—each one a dash of relaxation, anger, anxiety, love, excitement, fear or optimism. Part of your map right now relates to your experience reading this page, but there are hundreds more. Are you in a comfortable hammock or a commuter train? Did you exercise this morning or stay up late last night? Did you get a raise yesterday or did you get fired? Is your belt too tight? Bladder a little full? Gentle breeze blowing through your hair? If you take a moment to think of the flood of feelings that make up your emotions this instant, and then realize that there are massive, subconscious inputs that you're not even aware of (salt concentration in your bloodstream, for instance), you get a sense of what the limbic brain does for you all the time. The emotional mix of this instant, right now, reading this page, is the sum of all the individual maps you've generated around this particular experience, blended to create a single, complex, master emotional map of this moment in time. And it will be slightly different in a few seconds, or a few minutes, because your phenomenally complex inner and outer worlds will be slightly different, and you will have generated thousands of additional maps, and a different master chemistry of your mood.

Much of basic human behavior (not all, but an important part) turns out to be the result of massive automatic neurochemical chain reactions, and vice versa. There are also massive automatic neurochemical chain reactions in response to behavior—modulated to an extraordinarily high degree by learned and genetic influences, but powerful and inescapable.

The Dance of Life

There is one last step: modern life. Let's skip a hundred million years of mammals slowly building their brains, getting smarter bit by bit, and get right to you. Starting two million years ago, we began to climb out of nature. We started to leave evolution behind. Our brains exploded, tripling in size to create the subtle, thinking, calculating, problem-solving, tool-using, social-climbing, chatting, linguistic neocortical brain: the *thinking* brain. The *physical* brain speaks the language of sensation and movement. The *emotional* brain speaks the language of feelings and mood. The *thinking* brain, the conscious, thinking brain, our brain, *your brain,* speaks the language of . . . *language.*

Suddenly, in addition to our own brain maps of the environment, we had access to other people's brain maps as well.

Group-dependent, collaborative activities like hunting, forag-ing and sharing knowledge . . . teaching one another how to make things . . . took priority in early communication. Being part of a pack was good, but being part of a tribe, with real communication, was phenomenal: more food, better hunting, wearing clothes, using tools, taking a village to raise a child. In two million years, we expanded into every climate on earth. Language and the opposable thumb drove this evolu-tionary explosion, but only because we already knew how to love and how to belong to one another. Of course, cheating, stealing, lying and plotting to kill each other weren't that far behind, but they were *not* the primary, driving force. Helping, caring and loving each other were.

Now, with all three of our brains properly in place, we can step out of the evolutionary crucible and into our mod-ern lives. Free to think our thoughts and act our actions. Free at last, you may be tempted to think, to lead a purely rational life. Well, not quite, because nature throws nothing away. Remember that the basic biological building blocks didn't change. You just figured out how to wire the whole thing up in a completely new way to make use of the tor-rents of information that started to come in. The conscious, thinking brain was superimposed on our primitive and lim-bic brains, but they were still left with responsibility for a tremendous amount of what we do, how we do it and who we are.

We are primitives, we are mammals and we are humans, all at once. And the three brains are intricately wired to-gether. What that means for the limbic brain is that conscious thoughts and the actions they generate shoot back huge streams of information to the limbic system. Thoughts and emotions are partners in a never-ending tango: a dance of life, with no solos. Thoughts and emotions alternate the lead, but careful research has shown that, most of the time, our emotions are Fred Astaire . . . they take the lead. And our vaunted thoughts (in which we have such faith) are Ginger Rogers. Fred leads; Ginger follows. Maybe it "should" be the other way around, but it isn't. To make it more complex, our physical actions cut in on the dance floor, too, sharing the lead with our emotions.

If emotion is physically stronger than thought—and it is—that suggests a very different emphasis in the way we conduct our affairs. Cognitive therapy, the science of teaching people how to train their thoughts into more positive patterns, is as effective as medication in treating depression, and with a lower relapse rate. It's not Dale Carnegie, but it's not that far off, either. How you live, and how you think about it, is a big part of how your life goes, so there is a real premium on having *positive emotions*. The good news is, you can get them by *consciously* creating positive environments. You can do that by deliberately driving away the modern versions of lions and tigers . . . stress, loneliness and idle worry about status. By reaching out to good stimuli: exercise, decent sleep, rational diet, love and *play*. Happiness comes primarily from connection, from giving and getting love and friendship, and that's hard, though deeply satisfying work. Connect and commit, in other words, to generate positive emotions and drive away despair.

Dancing with Ulysses

Given the importance of the limbic brain, it's no wonder that you were touched when you looked into the stranger's eyes across the campfire, hearing his words . . . the sound of his voice. But the first intake of information to the limbic system, the visceral shock that you experienced looking into the storyteller's eyes, was just the beginning of a limbic dance. What happened next was even more remarkable.

Your response communicated itself instantly to the storyteller's limbic system. Every nuance of your response registered deep in his brain through his visual connections. The slight dilation of your pupils as the adrenaline hit, your shift toward him, the slight straightening of your spine, the flickering of your facial muscles as you absorbed and mirrored the emotions of the story—all fed directly into his limbic system. He absorbed these signals from each person in the tribe, and each signal changed him a little bit. Remember, this was all chemical. He didn't control it; it just happened to him. The tribe tuned in to him emotionally, and his response in turn tuned you further in to him and to the collective rhythm of the group. A great circle of emotion and chemistry formed between you and the storyteller and with everyone else in that magic group around the fire. And that circle has a nice name: limbic resonance.

Remember that name: limbic resonance. And remember the concept, too, because this extraordinary process does not just happen on special occasions. It happens every second that you spend with other people. Experimental psychologists have known for decades that we share moods. There are people who bring us up just by walking into the room; now you know why. You are always tuning in to those around you, changing their moods, and being changed by them in turn in a constant limbic dance. And the whole remarkable process feels good. Indeed, it feels so good (directly and unconsciously) that we cannot do without it. We wither, and we die. So do not underrate the emotional side of life. Connect and commit and be young.

Disconnect at Your Peril

L imbic resonance has its dark side, as does everything in nature. The drive toward resonance is too primal to ignore. Shutting it down is just as powerful as waking it up, but in a very different direction. Doctors and psychologists study misery and disease a lot more than happiness and health, so we know that isolation is the ultimate limbic danger.

After the collapse of the Soviet Union, enormous numbers of Russian men lost the only structure they had known. With nothing to replace it, many of them lost their sense of place, of belonging, of mattering, of simply being needed or relevant to their families and to their society. What happened? Within just a few years, life expectancy for Russian men plummeted from sixty-four years to fifty-seven years. They died limbic deaths. Heart attack and cancer rates soared, as did depression, alcoholism, suicide, accidents and violent deaths—all cries of limbic agony. In some ways, what happened in Russia is happening to many of us in retirement, and it's scary as hell.

Single men die years before married men: more cancers, more heart attacks, and lower survival rates with each. The angriest men have about four times the mortality rate after heart attacks as the happiest guys. Go home to an empty house after your first heart attack and you double the risk of having a second heart attack within a few months. Having close friends predicts survival, and the more connected, the higher the survival rate.

The beauty of connection is that it works at any age, because you always have a choice in this. You can reconnect at any age and reclaim the benefits of limbic engagement. Just as with exercise, you are always making a choice, whether you want to or not. Your childhood and life to date have a major impact, but even if they weren't so great, your brain is always open to change.

Consider, for example, the success of Alcoholics Anonymous. True, it doesn't work for every alcoholic, but it does work for many. A number of alcoholics have to hit rock bottom before AA begins to work. Think about that. What does rock bottom mean? It means you have destroyed all the limbic connections in your life. Everything. Family, friends, job, career, finances, home, community—all flushed down the toilet. Nothing left. Nothing. At the extreme, it's shivering, alone, in filthy rags behind the Greyhound Terminal, begging for quarters to buy white lightning. A howling, empty, barren limbic wasteland.

. And yet, for these people, there is a powerful road forward. It's a group of strangers who make room by the fire and share their tales. That's all it is: a purely limbic experience. Stale coffee, and too much cigarette smoke, in dingy church basements all over America and all over the world. But it works. It creates an instant community, a tribe, a group. And because the stories are raw, emotional and real, they are compelling. They shoot directly into the limbic system and begin the healing process . . . by reconnecting the disconnected. Talk about this to your friends who are recovering alcoholics. (You have them. If you don't know who they are, it's a signal that you might not be close enough to the people around you.) They'll tell you how it works. They'll also tell you that sometimes the meetings are a bust . . . and it's always because some windbag talked endlessly about himself without sharing his emotions. There was no limbic magic. But most of the time it does work, and it works remarkably well, because it's got a hundred million years of evolution going for it.

People who are truly alive to this are wonderful to know, and alcoholics who have managed to sustain long-term recovery are some of my favorite patients. Virtually without exception, they are deeply grounded and leading meaningful lives. Not easy lives—their families are sometimes gone forever, or so deeply wounded that the connection is always conditional; many never recover financially—but lives that matter. They have their priorities straight, and they work hard at them every single day. And guess what? Most of them would not trade their lives for yours. If you ask alcoholics who are really in recovery, they will probably tell you that they would not give up the discovery of meaning in their lives for anything.

For too many men, retirement and old age echo the limbic side of alcoholism; they are increasingly cut off, alone and desperate. But we can overcome the physical and social forces that push us in that direction. Most of us have friends and family, some degree of financial security and community. But unfortunately, we may not have a dingy church basement where a limbic group will welcome us, and that's the hard, hard thing about the society we have built. So our advice is . . . suck it up, be a guy and do your job. Build your own groups. It's not easy, but nothing worthwhile is.

Play like a Dog

Luckily, one of the best ways to build limbic strength is by playing. Puppies, otters, kittens and kids at recess are all hard at their limbic work. We suggest you devote a lot of time to playing from now on, too. It's a state of mind as well as a state of body, and it's pure limbic gold. Play with your friends, your wife, or guys you hardly know in a golf tournament or bowling league. Or play with a dog. Dogs are as limbic as it gets . . . not always that bright, but always tail-wagging, face-licking, happy-to-see-you limbic. And having a dog increases your survival after both heart attack and cancer.

Remember fourth grade, when summer was just around the corner, an endless time of sunlit days to ride your bike, play ball, read books and just generally goof off with your friends? Even if your summers weren't idyllic as a kid, you can have them now; our point is that you actually *have* to. It's not optional, it's not self-indulgent, it's *critical*. You have to use some of your time to build real connections with your friends for when life gets serious. So, before the bell rings for summer vacation, let's look at the serious side for a moment.

You may have a circle of friends who know you and care about you, and all you have to do is work at rebuilding the connections. Or you may not. You may just have some buddies—comrades, but not friends. They are *not* the same thing. It's why guys like war movies, full of deep and meaningful bonds that are strictly circumstantial. Work friends tend to be like that, close but not intimate. And like war buddies, you tend not to see them once the war is over, even though you may have shared coffee, lunches, late nights and the routines of the office in an easy and very genuine kind of friendship for thirty years. And there is absolutely nothing wrong with that. Buddies are one of life's real pleasures, and they matter, whether you're working, fishing, playing golf or poker. But you also need a few real friends. People you can, every once in a while, spill your guts to. It makes no difference whether they're men or women, but you need to be able to truly talk to them—and not only when the chips are down.

By the way, it's even more important that you listen to them when they need to talk. This is a skill, and not one our society teaches. In fact, many of us are dopes about it and start pretty low on the learning curve. So here's a little primer on the subject.

First of all, relax. Being a friend is limbic, with very few moving parts. It is *not* about solving problems, giving advice or, except in rare cases, taking on burdens. It is just about listening, and caring. That's it. Short, sweet and hard as hell for most of us.

Let me share an observation from years of practice. Dying patients invariably find out that a number of their friends disappear from the scene. I suspect we have all been guilty of this, and it shames us and hurts those who need us. It's not that people are terrible, and it's not usually fear of death, or hospitals or sickness, though that often plays some role. It's about feeling awkward. It's a funny thing, but the deathbed brings a lot of people back to those agonizing school dances, with the boys on one side and the girls on the other, and not a clue in the world about how to cross the floor to ask for a dance. People just don't know what to do. They are afraid to ask "How are you" because they don't know what to do with the answer.

In our culture, we expect a solution to every problem. Ask a question like that, and you become responsible for the answer as well. "How are you feeling, Bill?" "I'm dying. It hurts and I'm scared." What do you do with that, for God's sake? My immediate response, and probably yours, is that I have to do *something*. Bill is dying; *do* something!

Well, all you have to do, and all you can do, is listen and care. That's the magic secret of friendship. You usually don't have to *do* anything. You just have to be there and listen. Every once in a while you have to push a little bit with a question and the very rare piece of worthwhile advice, but that's about it: limbic resonance, no solutions required. For most of life's real problems, there is no outside answer that's worth a damn anyway. I'm dying, and I'm scared. That's a statement, not a question. You are not responsible for giving an answer, but you are responsible, as a friend, for sticking around and listening. It's a lot easier once you realize you aren't on the hook for changing anything. That's also all you need to ask of your friends, and you should let them know that.

We hope you don't wait until you're dying to build or strengthen your real friendships. Limbic muscles need to be exercised hard, just like physical ones. Your blood pressure actually goes *up* when you talk and *down* when you listen. So do whatever you need to do to share your feelings, and learn how to listen. Don't be surprised if you feel awkward here and there, and don't give up. It's a slow tide, but it's always there, so start swimming.

The last part of the limbic lesson is that being part of a group means giving back to the group. Altruism is a biological·need. You will feel good about yourself if you give back, and you will pay a biological price if you don't. You are wired for it, to give when you don't need to, so the tribe grows and flourishes . . . and so it is there for you when you need it.

The alarming news is that we are spending down our "social capital"—the willingness of communities to care for their own without expectation of payment. Meals on Wheels, school-crossing guards, civic participation, all the little things that make up a society. So whether you've stepped out of the economic mainstream or are still working and bringing in a paycheck, look at ways to contribute some social capital. Do it for your limbic health. You need to matter to the group. As you get older, you're often told, in subtle and not so subtle ways, that you don't matter anymore. But that's ridiculous, and you know it, so do things that matter. If you have a faith, go back to church or temple or the pagan altar of your choice. Coach Little League, drive a school bus, be a poll watcher, read to kids, volunteer at anything you want, but volunteer. You might not always like it, you might even find it boring, tedious or frustrating. Frankly, we don't care, and neither does your limbic brain. You need to matter.

That brings me to one of our more important messages. You have to respect yourself and value your life on a daily basis. No one will do it for you; when you retire, you won't get the social reinforcement you used to. So take pride in your contributions and measure them in limbic currency.

By the way, we think this road leads naturally to some consideration of the spiritual side of your life. The last thing either of us is interested in is preaching, but really, what's the point of getting older and wiser if you don't use the experiences of your life to ask some important questions?

So that's the science of emotion. Your physical brain and your limbic brain have a hundred-million-year head start on working together. Your human brain will never catch them, so stop trying. Embrace the fact that you have three brains, and work hard to nourish each one of them. Connect, commit and care.

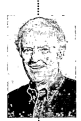

CHAPTER NINETEEN

Connect and Commit

I retired young, for what seemed like perfectly good reasons at the time, but almost at once I felt as if I'd gone off a cliff. Lonely, sad and deeply, deeply guilty. And bear in mind, I was happily married at the time, a ski bum, which I had always dreamed of being, and I was finally going to write. Besides, I had earned the dough to do it, so what's to feel guilty about?

As I look back, with the advantage of Harry's insights, it's clear that it was the absence of the old pack that was the problem. And the sense that I wasn't pulling my weight. Today I think that reaction was dumb, that I should have valued the long interlude of play. But the instinct to do your part in the pack runs very deep and consciously "knowing better" doesn't necessarily solve the problem. Even today, in the midst of an awfully good new life, I *still* miss the intensity of practicing law with a bunch of close companions . . .

hunting together, you could say. Loping up to the court-house, barking like dogs all day long at the other side, trotting back to the office, wagging our tails or licking our wounds. Working together into the night. The exhilaration of that stuff? Let me tell you, there's nothing like it, and I miss it every day. Not enough to go back, but I miss it every single day. And most of what I miss is the connection and commitment.

I wrote, I skied, I had various projects, but I didn't find anything comparable until Harry and I started doing this book. That was similar, in a way, to the old life. We worked like crazy, took pleasure in each other's company and had the interest and support of editors, agents and publishers . . . analogous to colleagues and clients in the old days. Most of all, Harry and I have been *into it,* as you can perhaps see. The intensity is its own reward.

At first, I was not going to mention writing this book as a form of connection and commitment. It's sort of pathetic that it took me so long to get started on something. And it's an odd-ball project, really, and not much of a model; not many people are going to solve their connect-and-commit problems by find-ing a partner and writing a book. But I got over my shyness when I realized two things. One, lots of people are going to struggle for a long time to find good projects to do in retire-ment. Two, and more important, mine is not as narrow a model as I had thought. All I really did, after all, was think up a proj-ect and recruit someone terrific to do it with me. Then we worked together like lunatics. The project could as easily have been a bed-and-breakfast, a community library or a hot dog stand. The point of it—the fun and the payoff—was the limbic connection and the commitment to doing something with a passion. So find a partner and write a book. Or build a new library in your town. Or open a hot dog stand.

If I were to fault my early retired life—not a very useful exercise—I would suggest that I had treated retirement as if it were a sabbatical or a long vacation instead of a new life. That's no way to treat a life that's going to last twenty or thirty years. Ultimately, Hilary and I came back to New York from the Rockies and basically went back to work. We missed our old New York friends and all that, but mostly we just went back to work. We still play hard and take a lot of time off. I don't apologize for that for a minute; I'm an old guy, I earned that right, and play is good. But much of the magic in our new lives is our work. These days it's writing instead of law, but the attitude is similar. I may be more of a project-type guy than you are, but do not underestimate the importance of connection and commitment. We were built for it.

Having boasted that we have finally cobbled together a good life, let me quickly say I still have a strong sense of how hard retirement and being cut off from the old pack can be. And how tough it can be to make new connections and commitments in the Next Third. But one thing jumps out at me: It was nuts to immerse myself so completely in my old professional life before retirement. In particular, it was foolish *not* to have other hobbies, communities and commitments— things I cared about and people who cared about me—when my work life ended. If you're going to do well in this country, you have to make a massive commitment to your job. No question about it. But don't make your job your *only* commitment, because it will go away. You need to get a life that will last a lifetime. It makes sense to start on that project as early as you can. Today would be good.

Here's another thing. When you finally do retire and it's a bit bumpy despite all your efforts, don't be too tough on yourself. Just as sure as there is a biological tide that sets against you at fifty, there's a weird *social* tide that sets against you almost simultaneously, stupid though that may be. So, you can be proud of any success you have—including the serious joy of just trying. In fact, forget about conventional "success" on this end of your life. The trick now, it seems to us, is being involved, taking your shot. Never mind if you hit anything. Getting involved in a worthwhile project, with people you enjoy, is its own reward. If there's dough or fame in it, good for you. But that's not what it's about. Harry and I hope we sell a gang of these books and that they help a lot of people. But if we sell only a handful, we have already been richly paid in the experience of doing it. That sounds so goody-goody that you may think it's baloney, but it's not. Trying counts. Connection counts. Commitment counts.

Cuddle or Perish

That is not how this chapter was supposed to start. Having gotten to what sounds like the crescendo, let's go back to the beginning and look at connection and commitment in a slightly more organized fashion.

Let's take a look at some wonderful population studies that drive home just how critical it is that we not turn away from society, not give up connections in the Next Third. There are hundreds of these studies, and they demonstrate the dire consequences of failing to live like the mammal you are. You can read more about these and others in a terrific book by Dean Ornish, the heart and diet doctor, called *Love and Survival*. His premise is that love saves lives. He's right.

First study: There was a famously misguided effort—early in the last century, when germ theory was new—to create a germ-free environment in orphanages. In the most advanced institutions, the foundlings were placed in aggressively sterile cubicles and never picked up or touched by anyone unless it was absolutely necessary. And they died in droves. In a 1915 study of ten such institutions, all the babies under two died. *All of them.* Being picked up, held and cuddled turns out to be essential to life. Love saves lives.

It is our mammalian character at work here, you will not be surprised to learn. It works just as well for rabbits as it does for kids. In another wonderful study, rabbits were stacked in cages up to the ceiling. They were being jammed full of cholesterol or something to study plaque buildup, but there were some anomalous results. The rabbits in the lower tiers did much better than the ones up high. Turns out the lab person loved animals. And she was short. She patted and fussed over the ones she could reach. *And they had 60 percent less plaque in their veins than the ones up high.* To check their suspicions, the scientists swapped the rabbits around, high for low. And the ones that were now reachable also prospered. It was the patting and touching, no question about it. Harry tells me that one has to be careful about drawing human inferences from animal studies, but my guess is, if you want less plaque, less blacky carbon and gummy sludge, get someone to pat you. If she's short, sit down.

While we're talking mammals, you may want to remember that *any* mammalian contact helps. A study of recent heart attack victims also kept track of who did and who did not have a dog. As Harry mentioned in the previous chapter, the no-dog people were *six times as likely to die* of a second heart attack as the dog owners. I sometimes get impatient with Aengus, our insanely demanding Weimaraner. But after I read these dog/health studies I went and got him a treat, which he took as his right, like everything else.

One of Harry's favorite studies, for a lot of reasons, was intended to see whether heart attack victims who were given medications called beta-blockers did better at avoiding a second heart attack. For some reason, the study also identified and compared results for men who lived alone and those who did not. The main test results were that men who did not use beta-blockers were significantly more likely to have a second heart attack. Not a huge difference, but an important one. And here's the interesting thing: The isolated men were *four times* more likely to have second heart attacks than their connected brethren! So what was the response of the American medical establishment? Almost all good hospitals routinely give beta-blockers now, but virtually no one inquires into, or does anything about, loneliness and isolation. After all, that's not what medicine is about. To which Harry says, why in the world not? Makes him crazy. One of the reasons he got so passionately into this book.

Loneliness is an amorphous and difficult thing to deal with, and doctors and hospitals are not trained for it. Not yet, anyway. But think about this next study and see how *any effort* can make a huge difference. There was a California study of women with metastatic breast cancer. They were divided into two groups, one of which met once a week for ninety minutes in a support group, for just six weeks, to talk about their cancers, how they were doing, and so on. The control group did not. The sessions weren't long, but there was intense bonding among the women. Not to put too fine a point on it, they came to love and care for one another. And guess what? The women in the support group lived *twice as long* as the women in the control group. *Twice as long*. Pretty big returns from a pretty modest investment in connection and commitment to one another. You may want to keep that one in mind as you decide about the social structure of the Next Third of your life.

It goes on and on. Studies showing that the lonely are twice as likely to have ulcers. Studies showing that unmarried men are two or even three times as likely to die of heart attacks as their married brethren. One of the great questions, it turns out is: Does your wife *show you* her love? If the answer is yes, you're in much better shape. So tell your partner you love her. Ask her to give you a pat, and you give her one. You both need it. You show me yours, I'll show you mine.

By the way, one of the best ways to get pats—and love, come to think of it—is to ask for them. I do it all the time. You don't have to deserve them, just beg like a dog. Ask my favorite question: What about me? But, again, it helps a lot if you show *your* love, too. If you hand out pats liberally, you get more. Same for snuggling.

Population studies are notoriously difficult to rely on. You can find one for almost any proposition. But there's no denying the logic of these studies, taken as a whole. Human contact, intimacy, is critical to good health. And the absence of it is devastating. Love saves lives.

This Society Makes It Hard

Retirement—being cut off from the pack—is hard. And in recent decades this society has done a lot to make it harder, not easier. Think of the big societal changes in my lifetime, starting with the family. When I was a kid in the 1930s and '40s, families were real, they were big, and they were very, very important. You knew who you were and where you stood because, most of the time, you were up to your armpits in family.

In my case, that meant three loving sisters and two parents who did not get divorced, plus a rich supporting cast of other relatives, many of whom lived with us at one time or another. My two grandmothers lived with us for a long time.

And during the war Uncle Ben and his whole family moved in, because he was hard up. (Pa was the successful one and just assumed it was his job to take everyone in.) Later on, Uncle Esmond, whose life wasn't great, lived with us for his last five or six years.

And the notion of openness went beyond immediate family. In the mid-1940s, a friend of Ben's, a funny New Yorker named Max Schwebel, simply moved in, for reasons that are still unclear. I think he had done something for Ben, and Pa was devoted to Ben. Anyhow, there he was at the dining room table for almost a year: "the man who came to dinner," we joked. Awful good company, though. And there was distant cousin Edward, a six-foot-five Seabee, who turned up at our door at age eighteen during the war and stayed after, when he was in college. Then there were all the relatives who lived nearby and were constantly in and out of the house. Pa's sister Gladys, for example, married Mother's brother Fergus. Think we saw a little of them and their kid? I guess. Oh, and dogs, too. Six big black Newfoundlands at one point. Plenty of cats. And a pig for a while. For the war effort, you know. The whole thing was a limbic feast, I tell you, and a joy for all of us.

If I could resurrect a household like that, I would do it in a heartbeat and never worry again about what to do in retirement. I'd just run the hotel. Cook the meals, call out the amusements and make sure everyone got enough pats. But that doesn't seem to be in the cards these days. One of my long-term projects is to see if I can't do something like that before it's too late. A handmade retirement community for some of our close pals and relatives. We'll see.

Another big societal change that makes retirement less cozy is the weakening of small city and town life. Towns like Salem, Massachusetts, where I grew up, have not ceased to exist, but the guts have been sucked out of them by the malls and the super-stores and the fast-food places. When I was a kid, a small city like Salem was the authentic center of its world. Locally owned and locally operated, for the good of those who lived there. We knew everyone, or at least Pa did. Cops, teachers, people in the stores and a lot of the folks on the sidewalks.

People stayed put more than they do today. My relatives had lived in Salem and surrounding towns since the seventeenth century, most of them. All of them, in fact, except for one courageous Irish grandfather who showed up in Danvers, two hundred years later, to revitalize us all. Today, I'm in New York, two of my kids live on the west coast, my sisters are down south and only two of my relatives live within a hundred miles of Salem. I'm grateful I left and lived the life I've lived so far. It's been fascinating and a world of fun. But I tell you, there are prices to be paid. Some of them are coming due now.

Maybe my family had it a bit thicker than some, but seventy years ago most people lived in towns and in families something like mine. And we all left. We just up and left. And changed the whole country. We left to start our nuclear families and move to impersonal cities, like New York or L.A. Where we could maybe make love to strangers or make more money. Get more stuff. And not know much of anyone outside of work and a small circle of pals. Funny thing to do, wasn't it?

Small wonder, then, that we gobble up books about traditional societies, like Peter Mayle's *A Year in Provence,* about a part of France where everyone knows everyone else and is in and out of one another's life all the time. Small wonder that we want to sit with Frances Mayes in her home *Under the Tuscan Sun,* in a part of rural Italy where the commitment to work is so much weaker and the commitment to family and community is so profound. Small wonder that we spend hundreds of hours watching reruns of *Friends* or *Seinfeld,* where the characters live rich, interconnected lives. We miss the connection of family and friends, so we watch surrogates, hour after hour, on television. Often alone.

Television is a little like those experiments where they put an orphaned baby chimp in a cage with a clock wrapped in a pillow . . . see how he does. And the poor little thing hugs it all day long, because it has a "heartbeat" and he hopes that maybe it's his mother. And because he's so damned lonely. We watch life on TV like that chimp with the clock in the pillow. Makes you weep, if you think about it.

All right, that's enough heartbreak; what are we going to do? Well, we're going to make a life for ourselves. No matter how hard it is. But there are no fixed prescriptions, no obvious ideas. And one size most assuredly does not fit all. So here are some notions, some things others have done, and maybe some guidelines. Harry and I are a lot less sure here than we are about exercise and nutrition. Not because this is less important. It isn't. It's just that answers are a lot harder to come by. The only clear message from Harry and me is: Work at it. Reach out to people and hang on. Love 'em as much as you can and get as much love out of them as you can. All the time. Because it's so damn important. And if you get any great ideas, let us know at *www.youngernextyear.com*. We'll pass them on.

Don't Retire at All

One of the most popular solutions that we hear about— and we recognize it's not available to a lot of people— is just to keep working at a conventional job. If the job is the flywheel of modern life, just don't let go. Whether part-time, full-time or occasional, work seems to give great satisfaction, even to the very old. Almost everyone who does it seems to like it. Not all, but an awful lot. And it doesn't seem to matter much what the work is. The other night, we went to a restaurant I've gone to forever. I said hello to Jimmy, the bartender, a nice guy in his early seventies whom I've known for twenty years. I told him how this book was coming and remarked on his good health and cheerfulness. Without waiting for the question, he said, "Work. No question about it. I don't have to be, but I'm here three nights a week and it keeps me going."

I forget where I saw the next piece . . . *60 Minutes,* I think . . . about a factory that makes it a practice to hire old people. Including some really old people. Works wonderfully for both employer and employed, apparently. The test of whether they're *too old* is whether they can walk up the steps. That's it. If they can walk up the steps, they can keep on working. And they do. I think the people who run that business are geniuses, and they should be imitated.

Same advice from a very different quarter. My law firm mentor, who has been one of the joys of my life for the last forty years, is now ninety-four. A beacon of energy and commitment and fun. I didn't have to ask him the question, either. He gave it as soon as he heard about the project. "Work!" he said with his usual intensity. "You have to have jobs or you'll die. I had to retire at seventy, but I've kicked around and dug up these projects: that environmental business [a pro bono suit to preserve the Hudson River], my little library [fund-raising and planning and politicking to build a public library] and so on. It keeps me alive. That and the boat. Thanks partly to you. I can't tell you how much that boat still means to me."

The boat is a nice story. He loves to sail, but in his mid-eighties he decided to sell it. It was getting to be too much for him. "You know," he said, "I could be cranking a winch and slip and go over the side." I paused for a few beats and said, "So what?" He laughed for a long time. And kept the boat. He still sails it all the time.

He is ninety-four years old, he exercises every day, he works his pro bono cases, he is full of passion, he is lots of fun . . . and he is not scared. He nearly died last year, some heart thing. I asked him if he'd been afraid. He thought a second, interested in the question. "No, not really. I was *concerned,* of course, but oddly enough it wasn't particularly scary." He shrugged. "It seemed . . . all right. It wasn't a surprise. It was just . . . I don't know, I don't think about it much." Later, when we were about to break off, he said, "Listen, be sure to tell them about work. I know you're big on exercise. I am, too. But work, a *project,* that's the thing!"

One of the hard things about the "work" solution, for even mildly successful people, is that they're used to having a certain responsibility that is hard to get in a retirement-type job. The work is not as intense, and there can be a fair amount of envelope licking. Still, doing regular volunteer work is one of the most satisfying things a lot of people do, and it does them a world of good. One study on the subject: those who did volunteer work once a week during the study period were *two and a half times* less likely to die. A study of younger women: 52 percent of women who were not volunteers had serious illness during the period. For the volunteers? Thirty-six percent. Dr. Ornish draws a nice conclusion: "Just as chronic stress can suppress your immune function, altruism, love, and compassion may enhance it." You have all read your Harry, so you are not surprised by this. But isn't it fascinating how closely our limbic lives are tied into our physical health as well as happiness? Limbic brain, hard at work.

There's a lot to be said for a paying job. You *know* you're appreciated when you're paid for it. And Lord knows, all of us are short of dough in retirement. Most part-time jobs are pretty modest, and for me it would be hard to get over my ego. But I think I'm wrong about that. My wonderful brother-in-law, a graduate of Harvard and a Navy Cross fighter pilot in World War II, is in his late eighties and is bagging groceries in Florida. He loves it. Loves the contact, loves having something to do. And is glad to have the few bucks. One of the nicest men in America, an authentic hero, and he's bagging groceries. They love him in the store. Why wouldn't they?

One promising area: the schools. They need assistant coaches in sports, and they certainly need mentors. One of the traditional things for the elderly is the care and guidance of the young, and we could all do worse than to have a finger in that important work. A fancy pal of mine drives a school bus.

Here's a minor idea that could be a major help: Learn to use e-mail. You would be astonished how vigorously my old, high-school classmates now e-mail each other, back and forth, on every issue under the sun. If television is an isolating and slightly toxic technological development, e-mail is the opposite. It puts a lot of people—including a remarkable number of people in their Next Third—into intense and meaningful contact with one another.

Have a Second Life, Using the Other Side of Your Brain

Personally, I think there is much to be said for not taking a job but making a job out of your hobby or your private passion. More specifically, turn away from your work life and your old work persona, and do something entirely new and different. If, for example, you have even the trace of the artist in you, nurse it along and live in a different world for a while.

I took that line myself, turning from the focused life of a trial lawyer in New York to being a writer in the mountains. I desperately missed my old life, as I say, but eventually I really got into the new one. I complain about loneliness, but my new "job" made life *interesting* to me in a way that another dozen years of the law could not have done. And that was true even though I was a pretty good lawyer and did not have much luck as a novelist.

I particularly like the idea of using a different side of your brain, different gifts, in a different part of your life. A number of us had to suppress something in us to be successful at something else. Many of us gave up the book or the painting or the study to be lawyers or businessmen or whatever we did. Well, take a look and see if there's anything left of that abandoned side of you. I have an investment banking pal who has become a good watercolorist. Travels all over the place to paint, and loves it. A lawyer pal is becoming a part-time guide at the Metropolitan Museum of Art in New York. Others write, and several have become scholars.

Going in the other direction, I have a pal who was a devoted mother and caregiver for twenty years, and she's recently decided to go out and be a shark in the business world. Not easy at her age, but she's doing pretty well. She had a strong natural flair, it turns out. And her successful lawyer husband is heading happily in the other direction, into a less competitive life. Seems to work. By the way, there must be a lot of baby-boom women out there who wouldn't mind giving commerce a shot while the guy tends the home fires and writes novels. Maybe not a bad change, if you can get over your stereotypes.

Turning to the other side of your brain does not necessarily mean the arts. I met a guy the other night who had been a corporate lawyer all his life. He looked it, too. Buttoned down, bald, steel glasses, the works. I asked him what he was doing in retirement, and he said he was working three days a week in a hospice for people who are dying. Asked what he actually did, he said, "Hold them. You mostly just hold them. And read. They like that, too." Wow. Not so many corporate lawyers hold you when you're in a jam, but that's what this guy does in retirement. He was not a boaster, but he was absolutely *glowing* while he talked about it. A little different from his old life, wasn't it? And it *nourished* him. It was new, it was different, and it nourished him. Like rotating crops in your fields. Rotate your crops. You'll get a better yield.

Make a Job Out of Your Social Life

There is a terrible temptation, in our sixties and seventies, to close up shop and narrow our lives. In most cases, retirement already does that, and it's tempting to just go along with the program, get narrower and narrower. Well, don't. It's killing us, for the reasons Harry explained. We have to "exercise" our social, pack-animal gifts as vigorously as we exercise our bodies, if we're going to lick that pesky tide. That means adding friends, doing more stuff, getting out there and being involved. And nurturing and preserving the friends we have. Same, of course, with family members. They're not all perfect, and we tend to get a little more judgmental and petulant when we get older. We're tempted to say, the hell with so-and-so. Well, don't; we can't afford to lose a one.

Play golf, by the way. It may not be great aerobic exercise, but it's a great way to get in touch with your pals in an idyllic atmosphere. The game is an endless fascination, and all the time you're pursuing that, you're also getting a limbic bath from your friends. People make fun of old boys playing golf, but that's a mistake. It is connection. And for many, a mind-enhancing passion.

Just Say "Yes"

There's a terrible temptation to say "no" to stuff as we get older. It's a hassle to do this or that. We don't really need to. Except of course, that we do. We need to do almost anything that gets us involved with other people. Because, as you now know, connection saves lives. So, until you fill your life up again—and maybe after that as well—default to "yes" when anyone suggests doing something or asks for help. Say "yes" to the dinner party, "yes" to the request for help organizing the potato race. Say "yes" to everything.

Simple example: A while ago I was asked to head up my fiftieth high school reunion. Well, there's a dull, thankless job. Besides, I didn't have the very best time of my life in high school and had not stayed in touch with many of my school friends. I said "yes" anyhow. And made a real meal of it. Wrote lots and lots of letters and hundreds of e-mails, made dozens of phone calls, and so on. Even organized six pre-reunion dinners around the country. Surprised myself. Met some new people and reconnected with some old ones. It was a lot of work and it may not have made much difference in the grand scheme of things, but I loved it.

Be the Organizer

Take it a step beyond the default-to-yes mode, and be the one who suggests stuff. Be the one who does the asking. You've got the time. So you be the guy. Start making the calls and don't get irritable because your pals say "yes" and then forget about it. That's what being the guy is all about. Keep after them, make it happen. You're building a life here. There's nothing wrong with the fact that it's hard. Of course it's hard. Look at the stakes . . . what did you expect?

All it takes is one person or one couple to make big stuff happen. Remember that bike group I mentioned? We're in our tenth year now, and it's one of the best things a lot of us do all year. It's all the result of an idea and a lot of work by a single couple. They thought it up. They made all the phone calls. They organize the food, the lodgings, the transport. And we go. Well, there's no magic to being them. It's just initiative, hard work and a touch of charm. Do it. What else are you doing with your time that's so much more important? Let me take a guess: nothing.

Incidentally, money is not a big part of all this. Organizing a bike group—or a cross-country ski group or a swimming group—is not money-intensive. It can be done at any level you want. It's the work and the drive that are hard to come by, and they're free. In general, there's little correlation between having dough and having a rich social life. After all, kids right out of college are best at it, and they don't have a dime. What they do have is a huge incentive— to meet and make love to one another. Well, you do, too. Maybe not to make love to one another, but to put together the groups—to make the connections that are going to save you in the Next Third. So go to work. Start a bike group, a book group, a poker night, a golf club, a political action group. Any damn thing. It all counts.

Another thing that counts is the spiritual side of life. Harry and I are perfectly aware of how important it is in your life and ours, but for once we did not have the confidence, the presumption, to take it on. And besides, that's a book all of its own, not a chapter in this one. Suffice it to say that a meaningful, spiritual life may be almost all you need. And it may make everything else you have a lot better. I have an old school pal who used to be a great athlete. He hasn't done a lot of physical stuff in recent years, despite my best efforts. But he does have a profound spiritual life, which is at the heart of his consciousness and his wife's. They're doing fine. I think he'd do better if he'd go back to working out, but hey, a spiritual life can count for a lot.

Oh, do you remember the second chapter of the book? The one where I asked how's your wife? Or your lover, or your pal, or maybe your golden retriever? Remember that business about loving someone like crazy . . . so she may love you back? Of course you do. Let me get back to that for a minute here. Because that kind of connection and commitment works awfully well, if you happen to have any flair for loving.

Let me repeat the advice in that chapter in the context of your new awareness of your limbic needs, and hers; if you've got a tolerable relationship, pour your love into it and try to get a lot back. If you're single, have a look around. Offer yourself to strangers. Link up. Rejection doesn't matter as much as you once thought. If you don't have a flair for intimacy, do it anyway. At this age, your very clumsiness is endearing. And as long as you're on your feet and feeling limbic, pick up a dog. Or a really responsive rabbit, I guess. Couldn't hurt. Or a grandchild. They're good, and they love a little nonjudgmental love. It's not your job to make them into decent human beings; their parents can handle that. You can just love 'em. As if they were golden retrievers, which they are, as far as needing and giving love is concerned. So are you. Get in there and snuggle. You won't look as dumb as you think, and you'll feel great.

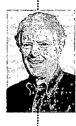

CHAPTER TWENTY

Things That Go Bump in the Morning: The New Sexual Life

Okay, here's the chapter some of you have been waiting for—with hope or dread—from the beginning. The one about your sex life in this Next Third that Harry and I say is going to be so great. Well, there's good news and bad news, just as always. And more surprises. The good news, I am pleased to report, is just what you'd hoped to hear. Most of us are going to be sexual and sensual creatures for the rest of our lives, making love happily and well, as much as we want, more or less until the day we die. Feel better? Good. You should. Things really are going to be better than you had heard, better than you had dared to hope. Especially if you do what Harry and I tell you.

We'll get to the bad news in a minute, but first let me call your attention to some crafty lawyer's language in the good news. We will be able to make love "as much as we want." Uh-oh, there's a hitch. The fact is that we will not "want" quite as much as we once did. Our libidos, which have made such fools of us for fifty years, are finally going to lighten up. The nutcase tides of testosterone that have made us unfit for polite society since we were twelve are ebbing. And you, you old fool, are going to be sick about it. Because you've enjoyed being a sex-maddened wackadoo all your life and think you're going to miss it like crazy. Well, maybe, but I doubt it. It depends on how you see it, when the time comes, and I think I know how that's going to go down. My guess is that you're not going to notice. Let me tell you a personal, disgusting story. The only one, mercifully, in this, the most personal and potentially embarrassing part of the book.

It's one o'clock on a soft May night in New York fifteen years ago. I am standing in a small, darkened apartment on the West Side. I flew back from a business trip to Europe this afternoon, went to the office and then straight to the long dinner from which I have just returned. I am fifty-five years old, I have been up for twenty-six hours and I am *ashen* with fatigue. Luckily, there is a bed nearby. Unluckily, it is not mine. It belongs to the girl who is humming merrily in the shower at the other end of the apartment. These are the closing days of my long, long dating life, and I am asking myself what in the world was I thinking when I begged her to go to dinner tonight. Her cheerful humming is a stern reminder.

She lives in a studio with a sleeping loft, which is served by a vertical wooden ladder. I decide to wait in bed. As I climb, naked in the night, I touch each rung with my bare body. Not what you might think. It is my round tummy. My round, tired tummy. Like Christopher Robin's bear . . . thump, thump, thump . . . going down stairs. Only I am going up. And it is steep. And I ask myself, like tortured Job, at every step, "How long, Lord? How long must I climb this ladder?"

There comes a time, sir . . . finally there comes a time . . . when we have all had enough. And we do not want any more. Not now, anyway. And we want to go to bed and go to *sleep*. That time will come to you, too, and you will just want to go to bed and the hell with it. And you will not be howling with regret or resentment for your fading libido. You will not see it that way at all. You will just want what you want. And you'll get it. How bad can that be?

Bear in mind, the sexual life does not by any means go away. When it comes up, as they say, it does so just the way it used to. And the event itself is often just as intense, just as much fun. And I am told, by Harry and others, that that goes on forever. *Nursing homes* are said to be hotbeds of . . . well, hot beds. Surprising but true. When my Uncle Fergus was ninety-four and in poor health, he wanted to marry one of his nurses. And consummate their already warm dealings. Happens all the time. So do not think you're going to have to wave good-bye to Mr. Wiggley anytime soon. He may not pop up as often as he used to. But he will pop up. And he'll be a world of fun. Same great guy as always.

Let me be quite clear on the good news side: I am surprised and delighted at how strong and pleasant the sexual and sensual life are in the Next Third. Like a lot of you, I assumed that all that went away. Or got so disgusting and embarrassing that no one would even think of it, let alone do it. Wrong. It's not disgusting. It's not embarrassing. When it comes around, it's the same old miracle that had us roaring with pleasure fifty years ago. Especially if you're healthy and in decent shape. You may find yourself making love in the morning sometimes, instead of midnight, to tap into your peak energy. But whenever the time rolls around—as it does with pleasing regularity—it's the same good stuff.

And when it doesn't come around, it's not the end of the world. Let me make a small plug here for the ancient art of cuddling. Harry is huge on this, for some reason, and he is not wrong. We are pack animals, just as he says, and physical intimacy is as good for us as it is for our dogs and cats. Touching is a primal and deeply important pleasure. Do it every day. Take your clothes off and roll about. Make love if you feel like it, but touch regardless. Make a job of it if you're shy. It's good for you. Or do it for the sheer joy of it if you're lucky enough to know how much fun it is. Foreplay used to be the slow buildup to the main event. Still a fine idea, but it's also its own reward. We are pack animals. Snuggle up.

Another tip for old boys: Slow down. Spend more time worrying about her. You're not in a rush anymore and she never was. Let's go up to the top of that hill together and have a look around for a second, before the sweet plunge. You'll like it, and so will she. If you were such a coarse, self-absorbed brute that you missed all that as a kid, do it now. You've got time.

Ready for some bad news? Okeydoke, some of us are going to have hideous *Erectile Dysfunction*! Just like on TV. Along with Senator Dole, and Mike Ditka, and a few million other guys. That's a real killer. The dreadful day when you *feel* like doing it but can't. We've all been there from time to time since we were lads, and no one has ever liked it. It's *awful*. And it's much more common for men in their sixties, seventies and beyond. Heartbreaking.

There is major help on the way, however, two patches of blue in that dark sky. First, all this aerobic exercise we've been touting is designed to improve your circulation. You remember that, right? And guess what? Erectile dysfunction is all about bad circulation of the blood to your winky. So, all

the good things you're doing for yourself in general by building a strong aerobic base go double for the sleepy lapdog. Get
his ears up in no time. His tail wagging and his nose wet.
Then, if that does not work, for most men Viagra and its
cousins do.

Actually, I've heard people grumble about Viagra, because
it doesn't make you horny. No libido kick. But that's wrong.
First, that's not its job. Its job is to make you capable, once
you *are* horny, and it's very good at that. And second,
because we are such suggestible creatures, it has a strong
"aura" effect: having great erections often makes you horny
. . . often leads to great sex. We're not here to give commer-
cial plugs to medical products, but Viagra and its cousins are
pretty damn good. There are kids taking it these days, and I
think there's a reason for that. After a while, just the sight of
the little blue pill will cheer you up. Make your mind a dog
dish of naughty thoughts. Lucky man.

All right, a different and graver problem: Suppose you just
don't care. No libido. What then? Well, let's talk about it. That
lack of interest can come from a lot of different directions. At
the slightly dark end, there are lots and lots of married
Americans who have not had a sex life for decades. Perfectly
healthy, normal Americans who once rutted like rabbits but
who just do not do it anymore. Not because they're old or
depressed or whatever, but because they just got out of the
habit years ago. They may or may not want to start thinking
about that at this stage, but that is not an aging problem and
doesn't come within the purview of the book. And perhaps I
should say—since Harry and I are always saying you *have* to
do this and that—sex is not mandatory for the good life. It's a
tremendous help, but it is not mandatory. Exercise *is* mandatory.
Eating right, too. And connection and commitment. But you
can lead a perfectly satisfactory life, if you want to, without

a sexual component. Not our recommendation, but very common and altogether doable.

Having said that, let us quickly say that sex is awfully good for you, all of it. And, within reason, more is better. You are now vaguely familiar with the notion of healing serums cascading about in your blood as a result of exercise and so on. Well, engaging in physical intimacy—with or without orgasm—triggers a wonderful outpouring of good chemicals throughout your body. Doing it not only feels good while it's going on, but makes you feel good in general. It is surprisingly good exercise in its own right, and it sends exercise-like signals in gay profusion. Not a cure-all, but not bad. And, finally, we were designed for it. So it's not a bad idea to get it on once in a while. Makes your coat glossy and flushes out your bad blood. Good use of your time. And your Darwinian body.

If sexuality and sensuality are so great for you—and they are—then maybe we should talk some more about reasons that people don't do it in the Next Third and what, if anything, can be done. Appearances count more than one might wish in this area. I guess that's no surprise, when you think of it; an awful lot of our concern with our appearance is a desire to make ourselves sexually appealing. So, if you think you're so fat and ugly and nasty-looking that you're appalled at the idea of getting into bed with yourself, let alone someone else, that's going to take the edge off your willingness to propose a dalliance. Self-image is endlessly tricky, but exercise and fitness can make a huge difference. Get in adequate shape and that problem may just go away. You're not going to look like a thirty-five-year-old model at sixty, but that doesn't matter. The trick is to look like a healthy sixty-year-old. As we said earlier, there is a world of difference between a healthy sixty-year-old and a busted-down old plop. If you're in decent shape at seventy or eighty or whatever, you're not going to feel funny pulling back the sheets. True. In this pathetic country, people go into paroxysms of excitement over even a mildly healthy-looking old lad. Which is a great help if you find yourself single in old age. And because of men's silly, silly practice of dying five years earlier than women, there are scads of women out there, looking for someone. That someone, cutey-pie, can be you.

Advertisers, pleasantly enough, are now pushing the notion that older is still appealing. They are putting more and more pictures of old boys and old girls in their commercials. It is true, of course, that they have ulterior motives; all you aging baby boomers have money to spend. But never mind; we are all being taught, at great expense, to think that older looks okay these days. Remember, when you were kids, no one over thirty was supposed to be trusted, let alone emulated? Well, look at a magazine today. Look at the movies. Think about *Something's Gotta Give,* with Jack Nicholson and Diane Keaton. Diane Keaton is deep in her fifties, and there she is with her duds off. Looking pretty good, too. Advertisers think we *all* look pretty good; I think so, too.

Here's another thing. Our tastes are changing at the same time. When you were twenty, the idea of making love to someone forty was a turn-off, remember? And darned if that didn't turn out to be stupid and wrong. Nowadays, I bet that you know quite a few women in their forties—and out of their forties—who look mighty good to you. People you would even sleep with, if it came to that. The sense of who is attractive, who is a possible mate, is a moving target as *you* move along and get older. It's not just a question of what's possible and who's available; your sense of who is attractive and interesting changes as you age. And older is more interesting. You don't have to worry about this, one way or the other. It just happens, but it makes your life more fun than you may anticipate.

I went to yoga class last weekend. Maybe there was some weird casting call, I don't know. But that room was full of some of the fittest, most beautiful women I've seen in a long time. Not just the instructor, Colleen, forty-four, who is the most beautiful woman on earth. There were lots of them. And it occurred to me, because I am working on this chapter today, that they were almost all in their forties, fifties and sixties. And these were *great* people. Great-looking, athletic and absolutely *going for it*. Not that I care, you know, but it's restful. It's restful to know that there are some fine-looking humans out there who are not kids.

One last zinger on perceptions. Do you remember when you were, say, fourteen and realized that your very own parents were still "doing it"? You were horrified, right? The idea that someone their age was doing it was disgusting, since sex was the exclusive preserve of people your age. The good news is that sex is still the exclusive preserve of people your age. And the age of whoever it is you happen to be sleeping with.

Summing up, we are mammals. We were born to make love, to play, to snuggle with one another. That's just how we are. We are *sensual* creatures as well as sexual creatures. It is intimacy, as well as sex, that we crave. Reptiles just want to mate. Mammals want intimacy. You, sir, are part reptile and part mammal. You have your cold, desperate needs, but you are also a cuddly little creature, built to roll about with your fellows. Our advice: Make love as much as you want. And when the reptilian frenzy fades, be a mammal. Cuddle up.

CHAPTER TWENTY-ONE

Relentless Optimism

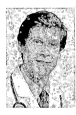

Harry

This has been a deeply optimistic look at aging—and for good reason. You have a choice in how the rest of your life goes, and it can be great. The rules are straightforward: Exercise hard and you will grow younger. Care about other people and you will grow happier. Build a life that you think means something and you will grow richer.

Chris has tremendous optimism about getting older, and he's right. The new science outlined here is radically different from what we thought a decade ago. And the lessons are pretty simple when you get right down to it: exercise and care. We've tried to show why this is so profoundly important . . . and why it's a biological choice you make every day. Our bodies are still part of nature, even if we're not, and they still run like railroad trains, on tracks of steel laid down over aeons. The train keeps moving forward, but we control the switch. We can choose left or right, growth or decay. The choice we make by being sedentary or isolated is as powerful as the choice we make by exercising or connecting. Remember every night, before you go to sleep, that you chose just a little bit of growth or decay today, and you get to choose all over again tomorrow.

Personally, I find the evolutionary biology of this comforting. I like knowing that I have a place in nature, and that my body operates according to predictable rules. And I certainly like the idea that I have so much control over just how I age. But mostly I like looking around the natural world and seeing echoes of my own biology everywhere I turn. Chris had to edit out large chunks of the book where I went off on tangents about the biology of squids, moose, worms, snails, fruit flies and bacteria. Still, the point is that we are all part of something much larger than ourselves. You are not alone in your retirement. You have all your ancestors on your side, rooting for you—three and a half billion years of family portraits hanging on the walls, urging you forward. It's a huge genetic retirement account that you can start drawing from right now.

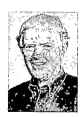

Chris

Harry is quite right about my optimism. We're finishing the book as I'm heading into my seventies, and my dominant mood is optimism about the next decade and, if I have a touch of luck, the ones after that. In a way, that's the most important thing we hope readers will take from the book: optimism about just how different—and how good—the Next Third of your life can be. My view of aging had been the traditional one . . . that grim arc of disconnection and decay I mentioned in the first chapter. With the experience of the last few years behind me, and an understanding of Harry's science under me, my view today is entirely different. And it is optimistic. For which I am so grateful, I can't tell you. It is a great way to look at the rest of your life. I wish it were going to be longer but, hey . . . I can live with this.

It wasn't that way ten years ago. Ten years ago, I was scared. Everyone, everyone, everyone fears and dreads aging. And the possible emptiness of retirement. And death, which seems all of a piece with the other two. You think about that little trio—emptiness, aging and death—all the time in your fifties. I certainly did, and I was still at it at sixty. I was physically active, but I had trouble finding a passion and I absolutely dreaded the notion that I would soon get old and sick and stupid. That I wouldn't be able to do stuff. Wouldn't find enough worthwhile things to do. Or anyone to do them with.

Today all that is simply gone. And it is not just an intellectual experience. Physically, I am more fit today, at seventy, than I was a decade ago. Stronger, more flexible . . . *doing* more. My personal life is fuller and much more intense, it really is. I have far more things to do and people to do them with. I have frankly worked hard at creating projects like this book and networks of new pals. As a result, I have more things to do—things that I urgently want to do—than I can finish in my lifetime. And because it wasn't always that way, I know what a luxury that is.

So here I sit, on the edge of my seventies, full of projects, curiosity and optimism. I believe I am going to have an interesting life, maybe even a useful life, in my very last years. I am not going to pass them in idleness, petulance and anxiety, which is the way it looked for a while. Not bad.

I know . . . . I may wake up some morning with a tangerine in my brainpan. Or ski into a tree. Fine. But I don't assume for a minute that I will be in radically worse shape ten years from now than I am this evening. Some decay, sure, but not significant. And certainly not debilitating. All the core dread about that is gone. And optimism and curiosity stand in its place. Not so many guys, I'll betcha, have gone into their seventies and eighties with those as their dominant emotions. And the bedrock of all of that is this lunatic exercise program, which turns out to be the only sane way to approach the rest of your life.

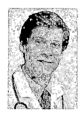

Harry

Exercise is absolutely the most important message of the book, because movement *is* life, and because it's easy to structure. Just make it your job. Chris, who is not a lifelong athlete, has chosen to grow a bit, just about every day, for the past few years. He has been steadily swimming against the tide, getting a little younger every year. At seventy, he says he has been sixty for longer than anyone he knows. That's a nice line, but based on his last stress test and physical exam, he's actually a healthy fifty-year-old today.

Most of what we call aging is decay, and decay is optional; it's under *your* control. Some of life's changes are not under your control, but this one is. Taking charge of your life, physically and emotionally, is the best possible antidote to standard retirement and aging. And it all starts with exercise. Exercise reverses the bizarre message our society sends older men and women that they should retire not just from work, but from life. The message that there is something unnatural about living a young life as you get old—being strong, fit, mentally and sexually active and emotionally involved. Well, that message was wrong. Growth and life are the most natural things in the world. Decay is what's unnatural. Chris is optimistic because getting into good shape has freed him from this social construct. It has given him the enthusiasm and drive to build a full life, physically and emotionally, heading into the Next Third.

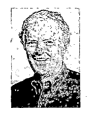

Chris

I passionately agree about exercise, but it's hard to overestimate the importance of connection and commitment. I was thinking back to turning sixty, a few minutes ago, and it occurs to me that my greatest fear then was not that I would fall apart—although I worried plenty about that. It was that I would be useless and idle and bored. And ashamed because I was not doing anything. When I first retired and found myself walking along the streets of New York at midday with nothing to do, I felt as if I'd just walked out of a porno movie. I didn't want my friends to see me, because they'd know I had no job, that I wasn't *doing* anything. I felt that weird guilt for a long time. In retrospect, that was silly, but I think a lot of men see retirement that way. We can't bear the idea of doing nothing, but we don't know what to do.

In fact, it's not all that hard, it's just unfamiliar, which *reads* as hard. Harry uses this wonderful metaphor about how career paths for the young are actually superhighways, carefully marked with huge, legible signs: GO TO COLLEGE. TAKE THIS EXIT TO PROCTER & GAMBLE. BECOME A USEFUL COG IN THE AMERICAN ECONOMY. But, he says, the paths of retirement are back roads or country lanes, with no signs to tell you where to go. Or who to be. No role models. No norms of behavior and no support organizations. In time, if you do it somewhere near right, you'll come to appreciate the beauty of the paths, their comparative calm—and the fact that you have so many, many options to do whatever you want. But it takes a while. And it takes some work.

You have to get used to the idea that, as with any meandering road, it is less a matter of getting someplace and more a matter of enjoying the ride. In retirement we have to rethink our ideas of success. Get over them, as a matter of fact. Most of us gave up far too much for success and got back far too little in quality of life. Eventually, you'll wonder why you spent so much of your life on that noisy, unrestful highway. Take the scenic route. And worry less about getting somewhere.

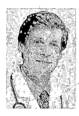

Harry

That's a great way of putting it, because building the complete package of a healthy body, mind and spirit is the real end goal of this regimen. Envision a new generation of very fit older people unlike any that has gone before, a generation living complete lives, with all the challenges, successes, sorrows and joys that implies. Actually, lots and lots of people are already living those lives, but they're hard to see because they're doing it on their own. They've gotten off the interstate, choosing to find their way on quiet, two-lane roads with light traffic. There are no traffic jams, and no rush hours. If you join them, you may feel strange at first, as if you should be back on the interstate, rushing along. You will miss some things about the old life, but this is your new adventure. And you will be just fine on whatever back roads you take.

There are only a few basic things you need for this new, back-road life. You need some sort of transportation, which is your body. Take good care of it, because it's the only ride you've got. You also need some company on the road. As Chris said early in the book, riding off alone into the sunset only works in the movies. If you're lucky enough to have one, wander the countryside with your wife or lover; if not, work hard to get your friends to share the ride. Don't worry so much about where you actually go; if your wife or friends have different ideas, let them drive for a while and see how it works out.

Finally, you need some old-fashioned courage. It can be scary on the back roads without a map. You might get lost—you *will* get lost, over and over again. The Next Third is going to be unpredictable. You won't have the familiar structure and support of the old life, but neither will you have a lot of the constraints and limitations. The possibilities are endless.

Our advice is simple. Forget retiring to an easy chair, with the remote. That's crazy. Work hard at the rest of your life, but do it your own way. Get into good shape. Then go out and take some chances. Get to know new people. Work hard at relationships, and get involved in your community or some projects. This may not all be fun or rewarding at first. You will take wrong turns and hit some potholes. But you will also have great adventures.

My father took up painting when he retired. He's been working at it for ten years and has had a couple of success-ful shows. I have a picture of his hanging in my office; it's my favorite thing in there. He also took up bicycling, after back surgery, blood clots and atrial fibrillation, and he is out there every day. My mother has written a novel, and she walks every day, winter or summer, rain or shine, despite having had her neck completely rebuilt. They work hard at staying in touch with friends and at being important people in their grandchildren's lives. They both grew up when FDR was president, and they are both still young today.

So take matters into your own hands, no matter what. Become the organizer. Take some risks. Build bridges. Some of them will fall down, some will be bridges to people you find you don't like that much, but that's fine. Some of them will eventually lead to real friendships. Besides, even if you don't actually like everyone in your pack, you still need a pack.

Build your passions. We talk about finding passions, but I think building passions is more accurate. If you have passions already, that's great. If you don't, then fake it for a while. That's serious advice. Pretend you're enjoying things, no matter what, until your attitude catches up. It's clear from research over the past thirty years that being happy is largely a choice. It's a decision *you* make in your limbic brain, with very little regard to external circumstances and with virtually no regard to money. Deciding to be happy may be the most serious commitment you can make for the Next Third.

One of the roads you should try in the next part of your life, if you haven't already, is the road to altruism. A lot of people have taken it, and they *all* recommend it. They set out to do things that help other people—most often in small ways, in little shared moments that added up over time. So give something back. It is a natural impulse and feels good.

Chris and I hesitate to talk about spiritual matters. Not because they don't matter, but because they're so intensely personal. Still, we both feel that there's a strong spiritual component to our journey through life, and it becomes more pronounced with age. As Chris quoted earlier, a life fully lived is also a life fully examined. That's all we're going to say, but we would encourage you to pursue the deeper thoughts when they come to you.

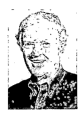

Chris

I agree completely, but good grief, Harry, we can't end on a note of sanctity. Let's make our last pitch a pitch for having *fun* as we close the covers. Let's leave 'em *playing,* like big children. They should be doing a lot of that now.

One of your nice points is that play is one of the great mammalian inventions and that it's good for us. Good for its own sake, without thought or justification. Because we were built for it, and it makes us feel nice. The reptiles and the fishes and the birds of the air, for all their beauty and skill . . . they do not play, Harry, as you wisely point out. We mammals are the only ones. And we should revel in it. We should tumble like otters in our terminal days. Snuggle like puppies and tumble like otters. Isn't that the stuff?

A lot of our advice is about "aligning ourselves" with our essential, Darwinian traits in useful ways. "Useful" is such a north-of-Boston, Puritan word. Remember the dreary sermons about "useful virtue," Harry, when we were kids? Well, play is "useful" in that high sense. It exercises our bodies and our minds in the most profound and useful ways. Play is virtuous now. It is its own reward. Golf. Now is the time for the boys to play golf. And poker nights. And trips to the ballpark to see the Yankees play the Red Sox. Time to go out in the yard and throw the ball, even if you stand twenty feet apart. Time to go tumbling down the bunny hill with your grandchildren. Race down the slalom hill with Cheeb, your seventy-year-old first-grade pal. Play in the surf after a storm. Throw parties for yourself, every single birthday. I had a beauty when I turned seventy.

Just plain *do* stuff. Default to *doing* stuff. Learn to cook. Jump into some new sport, now that you're fit for it. Just do it. Darkness will descend, Harry. We are going over the falls alone. But not this week. And probably not this decade. In the meantime, let us, by all means, *play.*

Okay, that's it. We're out of here. Last one over the waterfall is a rotten egg.

Appendix

HARRY'S RULES

1

Exercise six days a week
for the rest of your life.

2

Do serious aerobic exercise four days a week
for the rest of your life.

3

Do serious strength training, with weights,
two days a week for the rest of your life.

4

Spend less than you make.

5

Quit eating crap!

6

Care.

7

Connect and commit.

Author Notes

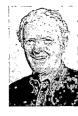

From Chris

Chapter One

". . . you can choose to live like fifty until you're in your eighties."

We sent some early versions of the book to friends for their thoughts. I was baffled when this line drew near-angry comments from two of the people I respect most in the world: S. Hazard Gillespie, ninety-four, my mentor and close friend for some forty years, and my sister Ranie Austin, eighty-two. Turns out they thought the book was too conservative. "Chris," Hazard said, "you make it sound as if the whole thing comes to an end at eighty, and that is simply not correct. Harry's Rules . . ." and now his voice gained some of the force, rhythm and intensity that thrilled courtrooms for fifty years, "Harry's Rules apply as clearly at eighty . . . and at ninety . . . and, I dare to presume, at a hundred . . .

as they do at sixty." Pause for effect. "You simply *must* explain that to people." My sister was every bit as insistent. I hereby passionately endorse what Hazard and Ranie said. The fact is that Harry's Rules apply with *greater* force and importance the older you get. Hazard and my sister are elegant proof.

Chapter Two

"Or your lover or your close pal? Whoever you got . . . whoever's got you?"

You may think we're tying ourselves in knots to be politically correct here, and that's partly true. But the more important truth is that *any* deep connection matters tremendously, right down to your golden retriever. No joke. All connections count; all deep connections count a lot. And let me reiterate, this book is not just intended for married folk. We happen to think it can matter more to single people, if anything. They have more decisions to make . . . more to think about.

Chapter Four

"Jump-start the sucker."

These vacations (and the "kedging" vacations referred to in Chapter Sixteen) are easier to arrange than they sound. My pal George Butterfield started Butterfield & Robinson, the premier bicycle travel company in the world. Write them (70 Bond Street, Toronto, Ontario, Canada M5B 1X3), or e-mail *(info@butterfield.com),* or pick up the phone (1-800-678-1147), and they'll send you a brochure that will blow your socks off. They command a premium, but they're simply terrific. Great exercise, super accommodations and meals, great fun. Take a peek at their Web site, *www.butterfield.com.*

There are super cross-country ski places all over the country. My favorite: Kay and Peter Shumway's Moose Mountain Lodge in Etna, New Hampshire. Among the cheapest and certainly among the best. Funky and glorious. You can write the Shumways at 33 Moose Mountain Lodge Road, P.O. Box 272, Etna, New Hampshire 03750, or call them at 603-643-3529.

For other ideas about biking, skiing and other exercise vacations, look at the back of general magazines like *Outside* or magazines specific to each sport. For less intense vacations, try mainstream magazines like *Travel & Leisure*. The woods are full of great places to go for a jump start or a kedge. Finding them is easy and fun. So is going.

"Do not delay because you do not happen to have a bath . . ."

Weeks after the book was done, I was sitting in the bathtub at the New Hampshire lake house, reading the autobiography of the incomparable Vladimir Nabokov, *Speak, Memory*. He mentioned that his father, a wealthy Russian aristocrat with democratic leanings, had been imprisoned by the czar in 1905. Put in solitary confinement, in fact. He said that his father had not minded it much because he had "his books, his collapsible bath and his copy of J.J. Muller's manual of home gymnastics." The collapsible bath rang a very faint bell. I walked dripping to the bookshelf in my bedroom, and sure enough, my grandfather and Nabokov's father were both working out with the same mustachioed Dane a hundred years ago. How nice to have that link with Nabokov, whom I admire so much. I am sorry to say that the regimen did not make either of our forebears bulletproof. My grandfather died of cancer in Salem in 1904, and Nabokov's father was shot to death by an assassin in Berlin in 1922.

Chapter Eight

"Building your aerobic base is the most important aspect of this regimen."

The fact is that "building your aerobic base" works near-miracles. Here's another bit of proof. Just as Harry and I were finishing the book, I did that Ride the Rockies bike trip over the Colorado peaks. Think about this: I am about to turn seventy, I am ten pounds overweight and my only training is the daily regimen that we're pushing here. Two experiences: I get a massage after an eighty-mile day. The guy asks if this or that hurts . . . if there are hot spots . . . sore places . . . on my shoulders, legs and so on. The answer, dear reader, is "no." No, there are not. Not one. And the rub-a-dub guy is astonished, because almost everyone has hot spots. The one and only explanation: a solid aerobic base, built up one day at a time for years. And good joints, built the same, slow way.

Next day was a hundred-mile pop over two peaks, which my pal and I did at a blazing fifteen miles an hour. We're out on our bikes for some eight or nine hours, including rest stops and lunch. In prior years I have been drained to a frazzle by doing a century at much lower speeds. When we finish this one, I am not tired or sore. I want to go out and have supper, wander around the town . . . boast to unlucky strangers. I could do another fifty miles, honest. And the only reason is this: I have a solid aerobic base and sound joints, which were created one day at a time with this program.

It really, really works. And it's easy, because you only have to do one day at a time. Then you get to go flying into old age on that amazing aerobic base, which is the envy of kids half your age.

Chapter Ten

"Hi, let me show you around . . ."

An early version of some of this material appeared in Janet O'Grady's *Aspen Magazine* in a piece called "The Sweat Shoppes of Aspen." Lance dates back to that period. I am grateful to Janet for letting me use my old material and even more grateful to her for publishing my pieces in the first place. I thought it was the best magazine of its kind in the country, and it was a treat to be in it.

Chapter Twelve

"The Ugly Stick" is my favorite chapter. As the older men among you will know, the list of "other curiosities" is a cursory one. If you have some additions, send them to us at our Web site, *www.youngernextyear.com*. We'll probably just lose them—happens all the time when you get older—but we'll try to run some for the edification of all. Do not shrink from telling stories about things that get better, by the way. Good news counts.

Chapter Thirteen

It has been widely pointed out by my friends that it is amusing to the point of appalling to have someone as irresponsible as I am lecture *anyone* on personal economy. I have run through a lot of money. And I am very, very ashamed. Well, sort of ashamed; it *was* fun. And I *am* more or less over it. But look, if you have any serious tips about living within one's means at sixty and beyond, send them to the Web site, too. We can still use some help. Not Harry; he is a saint in this area. But I could go off the rails any moment, and so could lots of other old boys. Send help.

Chapters Fourteen–Sixteen

Harry and I are fascinated by the topics of food and drink, perhaps because there are scores of lousy books out there on the subject and only a few good ones. My favorites are Walter C. Willett's *Eat, Drink, and Be Healthy* and Stephen Gullo's *Thinner Tastes Better*. Thinner does *not* taste better, in my view, but it tastes a lot better than you might think. Especially after the first couple of weeks. And it is worth agonizing over.

A story: Our old place on the lake in northern New Hampshire is a squirrel refuge; they eat everything that's not nailed down. But they have their standards. You know those virtuous rye crackers that everyone tells you to eat? Well, I buy boxes and boxes of them. Recently the squirrels found them and peeled all the cardboard and paper off. And did not eat a single rye cracker. Not a bite.

What do those squirrels know that Stephen Gullo and I do not?

 From Harry

The science of growth or decay ranges across many disciplines, and there are no standard textbooks on the subject, so the details in this book are drawn from hundreds of articles, papers and reference books. To make the science accessible, we distilled all that into a single, coherent story. It's accurate, but drastically condensed and simplified, with all the inevitable compromises that entails, but any errors in the science are mine alone.

That doesn't let Chris off the hook, though, because he's responsible for the book in the first place. He talks as if "Harry's Rules" were fully developed when we first met and he merely signed up as the demo model, but that's not the way it happened. I had been talking about the lifestyle issues with my patients and exploring the science for a long time, but Chris had been working on these ideas in his own life for a number of years before we met; he actually talked about doing this book together that very first day in the office. It took a few more years for the notion to sink in, but that's how *Younger Next Year* got its start. The science in the book comes from me, and the practical advice from both of us, but the experience of living it comes from Chris.

There are hundreds of good books out there on different aspects of healthy living, and thousands more that are not so good. We have brief reviews of all sorts of different books on our Web site, *www.youngernextyear.com* and will continue to add more as time goes on. Some books, however, stand out as core resources for living the rest of your life, and we have listed them on the following pages. If you enjoy reading, my recommendation would be to buy them all at once as a cheap investment in the rest of your life. In general, we are huge fans of books. They are dirt-cheap for the amount of information you get, and they are fun. If you find books you think are good, e-mail us at the Web site to let us know.

By the way, the same goes for great ideas or specific suggestions you might have for jump-start vacations, gear and exercise programs. Just drop us a line, and we'll put the best ones on the Web site.

Exercise

The books listed below are applicable to all sports and will give you a good foundation. There are good books on almost every sport you can imagine, so once you become passionate about a specific sport, read books about it—for fun, motivation and advice. (We've also listed a number of sport-specific books on our Web site to get you started.) We have intentionally not included a book on strength training here, because we believe that you need a trainer to get you started. And we haven't found a book that we think is solid enough to recommend for general use.

Precision Heart Rate Training, by Edmund Burke
(Human Kinetics Publishers)

An excellent guide to the details of using your heart rate monitor. You really should buy it at the same time you buy your monitor.

Serious Training for Endurance Athletes,
by Rob Sleamaker and Ray Browning
(Human Kinetics Publishers)

This is the bible for people who want to take fitness to high levels, like marathon runners and Olympic athletes. Surprisingly, it's very accessible, and you will probably find it both fun and inspirational. If nothing else, it will give you a sense of how far you might want to take this, so read it even if you don't plan to set the athletic world on fire.

Long Distance, by Bill McKibben
(Plume Books)

This one is just for fun. It's an engaging look at the ultimate jump start. The author, a middling athlete, had Rob Sleamaker take him through a year of intensive training on the same program used by the U.S. Olympic cross-country ski team. It's like a yearlong version of Chris's ski camp in Vermont.

Why We Run, by Bernd Heinrich (Ecco)

This is a wonderful look at the evolutionary biology behind running, by a biologist who is also an ultra-marathon runner. To my mind, he is one of the best nature writers around, and this is a great blend of science and story. If you like this book, Heinrich has written several others, and they are all worth reading.

Nutrition

We review a number of cookbooks on the Web site, but these four books on nutrition will give you a solid foundation to build upon.

The Okinawa Program, by Bradley J. Willcox,
    D. Craig Willcox and Makoto Suzuki
    (Three Rivers Press)

This is my favorite book on nutrition, and one of the defining books on how to age well. It is a look at *one* ideal lifestyle. It is not the *only* ideal lifestyle, and you are not likely to adopt it, but the lessons are important for all of us. The dietary recommendations make a lot of sense, and the authors do a great job of explaining basic nutritional principles. Read this as an educational book more than an actual program to live by, but make sure it's on your shelf.

The Zone, by Barry Sears (ReganBooks)

Skip the diet part of this, and read it for the nutritional education. It's a pretty well-balanced diet, and the science is fairly good, though not perfect. The real advantage is that it's well written, and Sears does a good job of explaining how to get good nutrition in the modern world. Don't bother with all the variants of The Zone, just get the basic book.

Eat, Drink, and Be Healthy, by Walter C. Willett
(Free Press)

This is the Harvard nutrition guide Chris talks about, and a great look at the best current recommendations about what you ought to be putting into your mouth.

The G.I. Diet, by Rick Gallop
(Workman Publishing)

Based on the Glycemic Index (a measure of the free sugar in food), this book divides the food you eat into three columns—red means "avoid," yellow means "use caution," green signifies "eat away." Makes it all very simple.

The Rest of Life

Successful Aging, by John W. Rowe and Robert L. Kahn
(Dell Publishing)

I think this is the most important book on the science of aging ever written. *The Okinawa Program* comes in a close second. I'm going to leave it at that, as a mild tease to get you to buy them both.

Aging Well, by George E. Vaillant
(Little, Brown)

This is a good look at several of the most important long-term studies of health and happiness ever done. These studies enrolled large samples of young people from different backgrounds in the late 1930s and followed them through their lives for over fifty years. The studies are not perfect, but they're by far the best of their kind and directly relevant to the principles in our book.

Never Cry Wolf, by Farley Mowat
    (Back Bay Books)

This is a classic, by a master nature writer, and a limbic feast throughout. It's a little dated, but absolutely worth reading and laughing over.

What Your Mother Never Told You About Sex,
    by Hilda Hutcherson (Perigee Books)

This is a great book about sexuality. It's written for women, but there are no good books on the subject for men, a lot of the information applies to us as well and very few men start out knowing too much about women's sexuality anyway. And the section on sex as you get older is especially worthwhile.

A General Theory of Love, by Thomas Lewis et al.
    (Vintage Books)

An intriguing look at some of the biology behind our emotions, with a very good explanation of the emerging science that is changing our perceptions of what it means to feel and to care. If you like the science of emotion, you will like this one.

Love and Survival, by Dean Ornish
    (Perennial Currents)

Dr. Ornish, a pioneer in the influence of lifestyle on health, does a good job of summarizing a lot of the research on the importance of connections and emotional support. This book is well worth reading.

How the Mind Works, by Steven Pinker
(W.W. Norton)

If you don't enjoy reading science, this is definitely not the book for you, but if you do, you have a real treat in store. This is a masterful look at the biology of the mind, especially the cortex, the "rational" human brain that we pretty much skipped over in the book. It can be a challenging book to read, but I think it's one of the best out there.

The
Younger Next Year
One-Size-Fits-All
Exercise Program

A s we hope you understand by now, this is not an exercise book. It's a change-your-life book. But so many people ask us how to get started that we've devised this simple outline of a regimen. Use it to get started. Change it up. Make it your own.

Level One

Your first goal is to do forty-five minutes of long and slow aerobic exercise without any discomfort. In other words, you should be able to get your heart rate up to 60–65 percent of your maximum and keep it there during a forty-five-minute bike ride or hike while carrying on a conversation. (If you've forgotten how to figure out your maximum heart rate, it's simple. Subtract your age from 220. That's rough, but it will do for now.)

At the beginning, do only what you can do. Try an aerobic machine at the gym—the stationary bike, treadmill, stair climber, elliptical trainer. Jump in the pool and swim a few laps. Take a walk. Maybe ten minutes will tire you out. Maybe you'll be exhausted after five. That's fine; quit. Maybe your heart rate spikes. Quit. That's also fine. Just get up the next day and do what you can. Keep at it until you can reach that forty-five-minute mark. If that means you're working out at Level One for the rest of your life, great. Just make sure you're out there six days a week, doing what you can.

Level Two

This level is not complicated. Do forty-five minutes of long and slow aerobic exercise four days a week. Do forty-five minutes of weight training—don't forget to warm up first— two days a week. Go to a trainer until you know what you're doing in the weight room. Then don't forget to go.

Level Three

Here's where you get to have fun. You're still out there six days a week, but you're mixing it up. Do forty-five minutes of long and slow one or two days a week. On your remaining cardio days (remember, you've got to do aerobics at least four days a week) go all out, reaching 70–85 percent of your maximum heart rate. Maybe you want to play around with some interval training, even hitting 85–100 percent of max for a couple of minutes, just to see what it feels like. Do weight training two days a week. You can combine aerobics and weight training on single days . . . but get out there.

And for your special Level Three bonus, do at least one day a month of extra-long long and slow. Could be a two-hour hike to your favorite fishing hole or a three-hour bike ride down a country road. Whatever you like.

But get out there. Have fun. Show up six days a week.